A SILENT BUGLE

by Sharon Cecelia Smith

A Silent Bugle
Copyright 2015 by Sharon Cecelia Smith

For permissions, please contact the author at:
sharoncecelia@gmail.com

ISBN
Softcover: 978-1-987985-56-6
Hardcover: 978-1-987985-55-9
eBook: 978-1-987985-54-2

Printed in Canada

This book is dedicated in loving memory to Mom,

who cared for and loved this man first.

Table of Contents

Part Two
Dealing with Disorientation   49

Part Three
Moving Past the Battle   81

Part Four
The Ups and Downs of Finding Help   131

Part Five
Finding Healing in the Journey 175

Part Six
Journaling Questions and Inspiration   225

Preface

In the fall of 2000, I started living alone for the very first time in my life. I had been married twice, raised a family of three children, enjoyed a successful 30-year career on stage, and earned a degree as a mature student at university. I had always lived communally in one way or another.

So to live solely on my own was an important turning point in my life and one that promised a chance to explore my own creative ideas.

The feeling of being lonely was challenging, of course, but it fashioned a need as well as a fervent desire to begin a habit of journaling every day. I had been introduced to a wonderful book entitled, *The Artist's Way*,[1] by Julia Cameron and a therapeutic way of writing what she called "Morning Pages." According to Cameron, writing these introspective journals every day, without fail, had helped her to find deep within herself an appreciation of life as an art form.

I took to this "therapy" with all of my being, because it rekindled a deep love of writing I had all but forgotten I had as a young girl. 'By the time I moved back home to care for my mom and dad, I was well ensconced in the joyful habit of writing these morning pages every day.

I would write fresh from waking, before anything else (except coffee) had a chance to influence or distract my inner world.

It is these journals, their insights, their spiritual questions, their frustrations—capturing the years 2003–2008 while I lived as my dad's primary caregiver—that have inspired this book.

Ironically, every morning, as I was writing, he would peek his head in my room and say, "Writing your memoirs are you?"

But it wasn't until he passed away at winter's end, Christmas Eve of 2012, that I became so acutely aware of their value, not only to me for the memories they sparked, but also potentially to others who find themselves caring for a parent with Alzheimer's and the plethora of conflicting emotions and behaviours that this difficult relationship spawns.

It wasn't an easy decision to reopen these journals. I was

aware that the nature of my journal writing during this five-year period had become cathartic, and, aside from a few somewhat positive poems, the entries were primarily desperate cries for freedom from my mission.

Sometimes, I could only read a few at any one time because the anxiety of my struggle back then, so evident in the writings, would surface as if it were yesterday. But, as I strove to understand what I had been saying between the lines, it became clearer and clearer how important this discipline had been for me. Over the years, the journals shifted and evolved to reflect the state of my mind or discipline of emotional thought at the time.

My world, every day, once I stepped out of my bedroom, was quite literally at the mercy of my dad's moods and demands. So this small space of time that I took for writing the journals each morning, before my dad was awake, was my emotional lifesaver in many ways. Not only was it away from his critical eye and solely mine to experience, it was also a healthy way to spew out the frustrations I could not tell anyone and did not want to act out on my dad.

For this reason, nearly all of the journals (except for entries from the last few months when my dad stopped fighting me) are focused on the problems of caring for him. These were the topics I needed to vent on in order to go on with a productive

Sharon Cecelia Smith

and relatively peaceful day with him.
And there were many of those.

Introduction

In 2003, at the adventurous age of 53, I returned to the home of my youth to care for my dad. As one friend quipped, "Maybe you are going back home to finish growing up!" I could not have known how right she was.

I remember my dad as a man who carried a charming and distinct air of dignity. Frank Ronald Smith was a Renaissance man—confident and masterful in social engagements and entertaining to the point of irreverence with those he called good friends.

He was also a great storyteller.

He would invent some, embellish others, repeat many, and

enjoy them all in the telling, as if he himself were hearing them for the first time.

It was a type of spell he cast as he shared his stories with the bold and mysterious magic only seasoned storytellers possess.

Though Dad very rarely talked about his younger years as I was growing up, as his dementia advanced, and he lost so much of his moment-to-moment recall, his long-term memory became very vivid, and his stories became biographical. He had favourite stories that he told over and over again, sometimes even 10 times in the short span of an hour's visit with company.

By the time he passed away in 2012, he did not remember these stories.

He did not remember who he was, where he was, or what was happening to him.

So lest I too one day forget, I am writing this story now.

My story and his story.

The story of our journey together through the experience of Alzheimer's disease.

Though it is customary in the realm of spiritual/religious thought to consider all of life's challenges a gift, I want to be clear that I do not consider this affliction itself any gift. And yet, the experience of going through it so closely with him, and the depth of prayer and insight it inspired in me, surely has blessed my life.

Since, as I have mentioned in the preface, I had been an avid journal writer for some years before I went to live with him, I had kept up the habit. By the time he passed away, these daily journals had amounted to quite a large box full of notes.

Some months after his passing I retrieved this box of journals from storage and began to consider their value as a rough manuscript. But again, because journal writing can offer emotional asylum, much of what I wrote was focused on my difficulty with the sense of isolation I felt as his live-in caregiver.

Now, as I note the various programs available for family caregivers who take care of loved ones at home, and as I have conversations with any and all who will entertain my questions and share their own journeys, I find a similar situation: the tendency for the caregiver to unravel along with their loved one is not so uncommon. In retrospect, I was not alone.

I am hopeful that by sharing my story you will see that you are not alone either.

I have included questions in this book for you to ponder and perhaps explore in your own journals. Through journaling, I was able to express and often purge many bleak feelings that arose around the experience. Over the years, the writings shifted and evolved to reflect not only my dad's development, but also my own. And now, in the rereading of them ten years later, I am able to see with a clarity I did not expect, how I did evolve slowly over the years in my ability to put patience ahead of fear, and dignity ahead of worry, and, most importantly, kindness ahead of rightness.[2]

This is the journey I wish to share.

Journal Entry: May 1, 2015

I rarely journal anymore.

I guess the need to purge difficult feelings has passed.

Or writing this book for the past three years has satisfied my need to simply write.

What hasn't passed, I discovered this morning, is the remarkable value of posing deep and sincere questions to my inner self.

And then listening for an answer.

For me it is helpful to put what answers come onto the page.

It's a form of capture, I guess, and a way of ensuring that the answer doesn't succumb to fleeting disregard or, heaven forbid, stolen memory.

This morning as I prepared to launch the manuscript into other hands, I received this response to a question I almost didn't know I was so deeply asking. I asked myself this morning why, really, deeply, *why* I needed to write this book.

The answer came so fast my coffee wasn't ready

yet!

One winter, a very long time ago . . . when my parents were still visiting Florida as snowbirds for half the year, my dad wrote two stories and sent them to my kids.

They were great stories.

One was about a rat that he found living under the Florida room of his home down there. The other was about a pelican with which he had a funny chance encounter on an ocean jetty one afternoon. Somewhere along the way in the past 35 years, those two stories got lost.

They got lost in the scattered momentum of my itinerant lifestyle. I didn't even know they were lost at first and quite honestly forgot about them. After my dad died, Victor, my youngest son, brought these stories up. Even as grown adults, all of my kids expressed a sense of hopelessness over this and a sadness for the loss of this connection to their "Baba."

The regret I feel has never really gone away in my mind.

Why did I have to write this book?

The answer came quickly and mercifully—that
I needed to finally pay the ransom note this deep
regret has been flashing before my eyes over the past
three decades.

Papa, I'm sorry I lost your stories so long ago.

We all miss them.

But look here . . .

Look what I have to replace them.

Part One

Identity Lost and Found

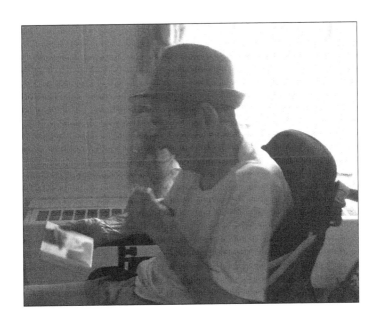

Daddy's Little Girl

Before I became my father's caregiver and constant companion, I was quite simply his daughter.

I was "Daddy's little girl" when I was very young, his "pain in the butt" when I was a teenager, his "dancing partner" at all the family weddings, his "pride and joy" when I sang, his "deep disappointment" when I divorced and left three children in his mind fatherless, and finally, when he retired, his "social buffer" from family criticism over his short fuse and frequent sullen behaviour.

He was a giant in my eyes, as fathers often are to daughters, and I aspired to keep up with and match his intelligent inter-

3

pretation of life and its meaning.

He taught me how to love animals.

He taught me how to love the outdoors.

He taught me how to recognize a gentleman.

He taught me the importance of being true to myself.

He taught me how to love words, and books, and how to read for pleasure.

He taught me how to write from my heart.

He taught me how to cry at a song and how to sing it.

He taught me how to rant against injustice.

He taught me how to hold my tongue.

He taught me how to fish.

He tried to teach me how to golf.

This is but a glimpse into the breadth and depth of the platform of values our relationship was founded on.

This is also a glimpse into the distance we both fell as his mind disintegrated and this platform dissolved into empty space beneath us.

His Story: A Class Act

My dad did not come by his classy ways through family status. He was born into a humble working-class Liverpudlian family. He came by it through his own elevated morals and outstanding intellect, as well as a desire, I think, to rise above his social fate. But he was not boastful in this and never criticized his family in any way.

His mom was an enigma to me as a child, sitting as she did day after day, year after year, in the corner of her sister's kitchen. She was unable to see and, therefore, relate to anyone in the room. Most of the time she spent mumbling and communing with spirits in the air around her. She had been like this most of my dad's life, and he treated her with great respect and tenderness whenever we went to visit on holidays.

I recall that these visits were a bit awkward, but it wasn't so much my grandmother's odd situation as it was the strange, almost secretive, atmosphere in the house itself.

The curtains were always drawn so it was dark, even during our daytime visits. My great auntie, who had not married after losing her fiancé to the war, was very sweet and soft-spoken, and she never lost her thick Liverpool accent. She looked like a child even in her seventies, because she had such a wee stature, almost bird-like. And she had a bird. It fascinated me to watch her float around the tiny kitchen with the little budgie perched calmly on her head as she served tea and biscuits on mismatched chinaware.

My great uncle, whom my dad regarded as his father figure, was also a mysterious character to me. He was not a talker. He also never married for reasons I was never privy to and had, as I learned years later, a penchant for the track as well as the bottle.

No one in that family liked to talk about my grandmother. After she passed, I was told that she had been studying to be a spiritualist and was a virtuoso piano and violin player when she very suddenly and mysteriously went blind and "crazy."

My brother is of the opinion that she had Alzheimer's long before it was identified as such. I'm not so sure. She was blind and mostly ignored in the corner of the kitchen for so long I wonder that she didn't disappear out of sheer loneliness. As a very young child, that was how I perceived her—sad and very lonely even though she smiled.

Years later after she passed, I learned that there was so much more to the story. My dad's dad, Fred, had been sent away from the family (for reasons unknown) when my dad and his sister were still quite young, and both children were sent away to another city and put into foster care. Another version that reached my hungry ears was that Fred, my grandfather, had caused a car accident that sent Jesse, my grandmother, into the state she was in, and that is why he was excommunicated from the family. Quite different versions of what really happened I'd say, so who knows?

What I do know for sure is that I found a letter written to my great-grandmother from Fred shortly after he and Jesse were married. It was a beautifully penned note, elegant and caring, expressing his gratitude for the blessing of his new bride. What I also know is that this brave woman Jesse, at eight months pregnant had crossed the Atlantic on an ocean liner by herself only a year after World War 1 ended, so that her son, my dad, would be born on British soil. So I know that, in spite of the family trauma around their lives, they were both quite remarkable people.

My dad was eventually brought back into the family and raised by his grandparents at around 10 years old. Gwen, his sister, was not the wage earner that he, as a boy, could be, and so she was not retrieved home.

Because my dad was expected to help with the household finances as soon as he was eligible to work, he could not complete high school. I always marvelled that he didn't seem to resent this.

The only regret I ever heard him express about his upbringing was the loss of his sister. Although he did find her years later during the war, she was not interested in reuniting with him or any of the family.

This bit of my dad's history was very important to me, and there were many times during my care of him that I rallied strength beyond what I thought I had, simply because he had been abandoned as a young child, and I was damned sure I would not let him "go out" the same way.

A Pugilist with a
Great Right Hook!

My dad had been a fighter as long as he could remember—
a schoolyard scrapper as a boy and an amateur boxer called
"Frankie" later on in his teens. He had been given this senti-
mental nickname years earlier by his grandmother after he had
been retrieved from the foster home.

He was his grandmother's pride and joy, and "wee Frankie"
could do no wrong.

It's a good thing he had her, because his grandfather was a
stern and unpleasant man at best. No doubt he is the one who
banished my dad's dad, Fred, in the first place, and sent the

children away.

Still, my dad never spoke harshly of his grandfather, but he sure did love to regale us with the story of the "Pugilist."

During the 1930s, while Frankie was an amateur boxer, he had gained quite an impressive reputation at the local city arena. His grandfather was absolutely against this activity and was fond of slamming his fist on the table like a judge's gavel exclaiming, "There will be no pugilists in this family!"

So his grandmother had a big trunk in the basement that she kept a key to and allowed Frankie to hide his boxing gloves there.

As much as his grandfather tried to instill an authoritarian fear in the whole family, I don't think he got far with Frankie.

Frankie wasn't afraid of anything . . . or any one.

He was a pugilist.

He fought anywhere and everywhere it suited him.

Even in grade eight, before he left school, he was always in the principal's office for schoolyard scrapping. One time though, he had defended his mom from a comment made by a bigger kid by knocking the kid out cold. It's not clear if this kid even knew my grandmother or her condition. More than likely, he was just a schoolyard bully, poking randomly at anything to get my dad's goat. Except, in this case, he targeted the wrong mom of the wrong kid and paid for it with a shiner.

And so into the office went Frankie, and, although he explained why he had punched the other kid, the principal had to administer the customary strap across the hands.

My dad, "Frankie," would end the story with, "As I was leaving the office, the principal stopped me and looked me straight in the eyes and said, 'I hear you got a great right hook son!'"

Every time he told this story his face lit up like a kid at Christmas. When he delivered the punchline, I would think about that principal and how he must have had a tender spot for defending his own mother to have said that.

Yes, he was a fighter by nature but also a gentleman in spirit.

One time years later, Frankie was in the ring for a fight when the other guy came out and just stood there with his gloves hiding his face and not moving. Frankie didn't know what to do. The guy just kept standing there covering his face. Eventually, my dad leaned over and whispered, "I'm not going to hurt you" . . . then left the ring losing the bout by default.

He told that story hundreds of times, a look of delightful puzzlement on his face with every telling.

Journal Entry: November 16, 2004

I wish I could walk away because it's so distressing, and I feel so very alone.

I need an intervention of some kind; God knows because I am not a fighter.

I do not want to be the opponent, the one who stands out as the victim of my dad's pent up rage.

Everyone in the family seems to be sitting on the sideline waiting for me to take that role.

Or for a disaster to happen.

But no doubt I would be assigned the blame in that too! —Still in centre ring alone.

I don't want to fight any more.

How can I avoid being my dad's verbal punching bag, so to speak, and still keep him safe?

I know he can't help it.

Frankie Was Always a Bit of a Lone Marcher

My dad was in the Air Force marching band in Ottawa during World War II.

He was a bugler.

One of my mom's favourite stories was of a time when they were dating, and, during one of the marching exercises, my dad's mind was not on the marching duty at hand but rather blissfully recalling his sweetheart back home.

As the marching corps made its way through the streets of Ottawa, they turned a corner in perfect synchronized form and continued along a new path.

All of the players, that is, except Frankie.

He was always a bit of a lone marcher, but this was quite literal.

There he was, marching all by himself straight on down the street, daydreaming away, looking like a very silly fellow indeed!

As the story goes, he earned KP duty (Kitchen Patrol, which usually means peeling potatoes) for this disrespectful display of inattention.

I don't think he cared much, though.

He married that sweetheart, my mom, in 1942 before the war was even over.

He just loved to amuse us with this story of her bewitching power over him. I think he enjoyed the blush it brought to her cheeks every time.

I Did Not Take His Behaviour Personally ... Or Did I?

Of all the people in the world who are looking after a parent or other family elder with Alzheimer's, I think I am the last one who should be writing a book. In my own humble opinion, looking back now, I don't think I was all that good at it. I made every mistake there was to make and invented a few along the way.

I came to the mission, as it were, involuntarily and less than qualified personality-wise. Oh, I had worked for years as a professional caregiver in nursing homes as well as private residences, and I was hoping that that experience had prepared me to be a full-time caregiver to my dad. I had been good in this line of work, because of the gentle way I had with the residents. They were so frail and vulnerable that they brought out the easygoing, patient side of my character.

But, holy smokes, my dad was a whole different kettle of fish! It took longer than I care to admit for me to access some of this same caring composure with him.

We were so similar he and I. We both tended to be impatient, stubborn, hotheaded, and critical. And when his mood swings ignited these negative tendencies in him, I too displayed very similar traits. I'd get impatient at his impatience, bullheaded when he resisted my help, snappy and resentful with his intolerant opinions.

Even though I was aware of this tendency, the clash could happen so fast!

I see now how important the journaling had been for me in this regard. I needed that outlet to release my frustrations and irritability so that I could care for him with a professional objectivity. A purely personal level of caring could so easily get tangled with my own feelings.

In the end though, I feel that I did work hard to overcome my own impulsive reactions to the behaviours this tragic illness creates. Because above, around, and beneath the struggle was a firm foundation of love. The pure and simple truth is I loved my dad like crazy, and so I "kept on keepin' on," as they say, mistakes and all.

An Alzheimer's Daughter

I knew the illness was the cause of much of his discontent and anger, and I knew he wasn't meaning to lash out at me. I knew this not only from working with other dementia patients but also from my years as his precious daughter, whom he cherished and loved dearly and openly.

I also knew that the illness was the cause of his constant suspiciousness and compulsive fault-finding with everything. This too was a deep knowing from a life lived with him as a fair and encouraging teacher as well as a father.

I tried not to take his behaviour personally, but it is difficult not to revert back to being a child, accepting the judgment of the parent. And, in spite of my mature age, I spent some of the time emotionally hijacked by that role.

After all, I was so familiar with it.

It was a role I think I literally craved as time measured out his disappearance in my life.

And that is the paradox, isn't it? The paradox that still stings. He was not disappearing from my life, he was disappearing while still in it.

When I could not be his daughter because he wasn't there, I remained in his life as a daughter anyway, even if to the illness itself in the end.

But as much as I may have succeeded as his daughter in not taking his behaviours personally, I definitely took the affront of the illness itself that way.

I took it personally on behalf of my dad, because he couldn't.

I took it personally that this dreadful illness was robbing me of someone I loved right before my eyes.

I took it personally that it didn't matter how hard I tried to hold on to him, this thief called Alzheimer's was going to win.

I took it personally that he couldn't see how I was helping him and know it was because I loved him, because he was loved.

As an Alzheimer's daughter, I took it damn personally.

This caused much of my struggle, I know. Fortunately, the many roles I fulfilled apart from being a daughter helped me weather the storms of this contradiction.

When, as a daughter, I felt besieged by the experience, I could draw upon these abilities:

- As a mother I knew how to be instinctively protective and kind.
- As a friend I knew how to be fiercely loyal and honest.
- As an artist I knew it was important to keep creative expression in my life, which is why I wrote every day.

I am so very grateful to these aspects of my own nature for having my back when I felt weak and needed strength. But I am particularly thankful for the creative impulse that sustained that faithful habit of journaling. It served so many purposes aside from the therapeutic purge of troublesome emotions. It helped me to nurture my more complete identity, to recall a memory when I felt overwhelmed, or to create a poem when I felt depleted, and, ultimately, to inspire an insight when I felt lost.

Journal Entry: August 28, 2005

I hope there are morning glories in heaven.

They sooth my soul so completely.

All I can think of these days is to take one day at a time.

I honestly thought I had passed a portal of some kind into a new level of patience and kindness.

But my dad is driving me nuts again.

I am trying so hard to change, and he just can't.

Don't know why I expect him to, for goodness' sake.

He was stubborn before he even got this damn illness.

Why would he suddenly become un-stubborn?

Seriously, my attitude is worse than his some days.

I know it is not him I'm pissed off with.

It's this damn dementia.

But he feels the anger anyway like he is to blame.

And then gets defensive.

Bad circle for sure.

Journal Entry: April 22, 2009

Well, today I'm feeling pretty good.

I surprised myself last night when Dad told me I should be ashamed of myself.

He means for putting him in a home, I guess.

I didn't feel ashamed.

Which is a big deal.

It has taken me five years to finally not allow my initial child response to be the voice I listen to.

Slow learner but learner nonetheless.

It still hurts when he says these things but not like before.

Now it just hurts because I know it's not him talking.

It hurts that some other voice is using my dad.

But, I didn't let it spoil our visit, so there.

I feel good today.

Who Is an Alzheimer's Sufferer?

As Alzheimer's advances, so does the unpredictability of everything.

My dad could change tack abruptly, one moment being unreasonably aggressive and the next moment sweet as apple pie. He would usually have no awareness that this had happened. This was upsetting to me, because I was not always able to let go of the turmoil he had created between us quite as quickly as he had.

This, of course, begs the question: Who is the real sufferer in the course of this disease?

It is a form of suffering that we may not expect. It may take us wholly by surprise, because, like Alzheimer's, it is dictated by an unpredictability that we can brace for, but are never really prepared for.

One of the great rewards of my discipline of journaling was that I could vent my feelings about my own struggles in the writings and not at my dad.

Most of the time, that is.

My Dad had such a strong mind, such a clever mind, that, at the end, when the deterioration was extreme and his aggression escalated into flailing and such, he could suddenly come clear at the end of a bout of crazy-eyed boxing at the nurses, look up at them teary-eyed and say, "Did I hit you? I'm sorry, honey."

It touched their hearts, but it broke mine.

That was a whole different level of suffering.

For my dad and for me.

I knew that somewhere, somehow he knew.

And so we both became helpless victims.

Journal Entry: January 13, 2005

What's wrong with me?

It's an expression I heard many times growing up.

It came out of my dad's mouth.

Now I hear it coming out of mine.

I understand that my dad's moods and behaviours are not always within his conscious control.

But I still have moments of frustration and annoyance as if he can control these things, as if he misbehaves on purpose to bug me.

One minute, he is Mr. Nasty, and the next minute, literally the next minute, he turns into Prince Charming!

But, there I am still processing the verbal abuse of Mr. Nasty!

I know that my frustration only confuses him, so I try not to let it show.

I know he lives in an exaggerated state of mind much of the time, but why do I have to feel like shit too?

I used to think my liberal beliefs kept my mind flexible and open to change.

But this is a merciless lesson, God.

As if his mental collapse isn't enough, now I have to deal with this fault line in my own mental makeup.

I need a lifeline here.

Tyler Bar the Gates!

No matter where he went, or who was there, my dad was easily the funniest person in the room.

A ham at heart, he commanded an audience as naturally as most of us breathe and rarely disappointed once he had everyone's rapt attention.

One story, as told by one of his Masonic Lodge brethren, never fails to make me smile.

My dad belonged to a rather stodgy suburban lodge called St. Andrew's Lodge in the 1970s, and he took his duties very seriously, having risen to the rank of Worshipful Master.

However, one evening he took his seat in the East, (masonic

terminology for the head table) then suddenly rose, banging his gavel on the podium loudly, declaring, "Tyler bar the gates!"

The lodge went silent.

All members snapped up in their seats and gave their respectful attention to the revered leader.

Now, in conventional Lodge behaviour, one would only summon the Tyler (the ceremonial protector of the gathering) like that if a rather serious matter was about to be discussed: a matter of moral or even legal protocol.

My dad continued. "I cannot find my glasses."

As the room started to rustle with collective disbelief, he went for the gusto and rose to his feet once again, now waving his "found" glasses and declaring in masterful fashion, "Tyler un-bar the gates!"

No one had ever done something like this in the Lodge before.

Taken out of the context of my Dad's great ability with humour, this would *not* have been received well. But, as his fate would have it, the room broke up laughing, and, as my brother Ron (also a mason) likes to say, "The walls came tumbling down."

According to Ron, the lodge attendance increased dramatically when our dad was in that seat. Brethren came in anticipation of what the Master would say next, and not out of a dull sense of duty. Lodge became a place of enjoyment and cama-raderie. In fact, he was asked to hold the title of Lodge Master for two terms in a row, something that had not occurred in that Masonic community since the 1800s!

Everywhere he went, people were moved by his authentic nature and the rich fearlessness with which he shared it. Even later, at the height of his captivity to Alzheimer's he would un-expectedly retrieve this grand humour and treat whoever was in earshot to a moment's delight.

When it was finally necessary for him to enter a nursing home, rarely would I go to see him when one of the staff did not seek me out to share something unique and comical of the day's adventures with him.

I am so grateful today as I look back on these years with my dad that he had this advanced sense of humour. Even though it was as unpredictable as the other aspects of his character at this time, it worked well that way. The suddenness of his playful and jovial outbursts were like flash rains in an otherwise withering situation. Even if the quips were ones I had heard before, his delivery was always refreshing and entertaining.

On a number of occasions, I have been told that I inher-ited my dad's sense of humour. I smile and express thanks for the compliment, of course, but secretly I'm thinking, "Not even close!"

As much as I struggled and even suffered because of his illness, I was redeemed so many more times by this remarkable side of his nature.

Many were.

Even when there was so little left to give, he managed to squeeze out a chuckle for someone.

The Trickster Backfires

My dad possessed a wonderful sense of respect when it came to his cheeky imagination and the protocol of whatever situation he was in. He knew when to pull back his decidedly irreverent behaviour in the nick of time, and he was never crass in the presence of women or children. My brother does confess, however, that this discrimination was modified when it was just the men and boys alone.

There was this one time, though.

He always told this story with subdued laughter and a look of chagrin on his face. My dad's last job before retiring was as the chief industrial engineer for a small lighting company. As such, he was one of the head honchos in the firm, and the owner was quite fond of him as a person. The summer he was hired, he accompanied a few chosen members of the executive to attend a business retreat weekend at the boss's cottage. Being new to the team, he behaved himself well enough, but, on the third day, the sun and surf part of the weekend apparently brought out adolescent memories and consequently his own carefree behaviour.

As the story goes, the other gentlemen were lounging on the dock one afternoon when my dad was coming in from a solo canoe paddle around the lake, and a mischievous spirit overtook him. He suddenly tipped the canoe over, pretending, of course, that it was an accident. Then, without surfacing, he swam under the overturned canoe and up into the pocket of air that he knew existed there. Here he safely tread water, all the while stifling a belly laugh and thoroughly enjoying the kerfuffle his little gag was sure to create on the dock.

At first, the voices erupted in a chorus of cheers and sneers, but, after a few minutes, a strange and heavy silence hovered in the air.

It wasn't so funny anymore.

Something was wrong; something was off.

Fear quickly filled the air.

Well, something was off alright, and unfortunately it turned out to be Frankie's timing. He stayed under the canoe two seconds too long, because as his head finally broke the water's surface with an unabashed grin filling his face, it became painfully obvious that he was alone in his appreciation of the joke. He was immediately summoned to the cottage by his new boss and reprimanded severely.

As my dad told it, he was lucky to still have a job after that weekend.

As I tell it, he was just proving once again that he had some kind of season's pass from the price most of us pay for misbehaving, because he was just so damn likeable.

Is This Me?

I know that it is not uncommon for personal possessions to appear or disappear from the room(s) of a person living with Alzheimer's, whether by their own hand or that of a roommate. It did seem with my dad, though, that many of the mysterious "acquisitions" became pivotal pieces of the puzzle for me, often giving me profound pause for thought in my own desire to find peace within the chaos, revelation within the absurd.

He had a hat, a fedora, that had suddenly appeared in his room one day from out of nowhere, and since no one in the home seemed to know whose it was, he just kept wearing it. It was clean and in good shape and looked very jaunty perched on his head, so I let him continue to wear it.

When he became unable to enjoy watching TV because of failing eyesight, I set up a CD player in his room so he could enjoy music. My daughter had brought in a CD collection of Frank Sinatra's best hits, and it played constantly.

One day, I came in, and there he was with the hat on sitting in rapt attention, staring at the CD cover and listening intently to the crooner's voice.

The picture on the CD cover was one of Sinatra in a fedora.

It was uncanny, really.

As a young man, my dad had been remarkably handsome, a very fashionable dresser in his zoot suits, and on top of it all a beautiful singer. Still now, he looked strikingly like this picture (albeit quite a bit older) in his jaunty mystery hat. As I stood there silently watching him enjoying the song, he suddenly realized I was there, looked up, and said to me, "Is this me?"

"Yes," I said, the musician in me not skipping a single beat. "Boy oh boy, could you sing, eh?"

Then we just continued to listen together to "Sweet Lorraine."

It was beautiful and surreal at the same time.

Was I in his world then?

From Dad to Papa

Somewhere along the way, I stopped calling my dad, *Dad*. I had been calling him Dad all my life, and, except for the era of the Frankie stories when we all called him Frankie now and again, I had never thought of him as anything but Dad.

But, in about the third year of our journey together, I suddenly found myself calling him Papa. The word just appeared from out of nowhere, it seemed, and became a common part of our rapport.

I liked the soft sweet sound of it. It made *me* feel softer and sweeter in turn.

There was a soothing kindness to the way it rolled out of

my mouth.

My dad never objected to it, so I just assumed it made him feel good, too.

Something about the earthy ethnicity of the word itself lifted us both out of the mundane sameness of plain old official sounding *Dad* and gave our relationship a sense of continuity, of ancestral significance. At least, for me it did, so I continued to call him that for the last few years of our time together.

Then again, I just may have unconsciously adopted it because of my fondness for the song "Papa, Can You Hear Me?" from the Broadway hit musical *Yentle*. I had long admired the way Streisand sang that song so tenderly, and fancying myself as the heroine in a musical could have had the potential to empower my weakening resolve.

But, in all seriousness, it was that feeling of tenderness that was so vital for me. I think the tenderness of the word *Papa* alone helped me cope with and relinquish my own stubborn resistance to losing what he had been in order to gently accept what he was becoming.

A Man and His Dog

Along with the hat and the word *Papa* that appeared out of nowhere, on another day, some time later, came a dog. A little stuffed, Yorkie kind of dog.

How did it get into his room? It wasn't new, so no one brought it as a gift.

It just showed up.

For the first while, it seemed my dad knew this dog was a stuffed toy. He regarded it at the end of his bed with a certain detachment. Then, in the last winter of his life, when he became less and less able to rise from his bed, that changed.

This little stuffed Yorkie took on life.

The nurses went along with the new boarder in his room and washed it and fed it (or so they told him so *he* wouldn't feed it so much). It was never far from his petting hand and seemed quite the content little canine staring stiffly out the window all day long.

I never referred to this dog by any name in particular, and Dad never offered one. We all just called it "your dog," and that seemed to please him. He had been a dog-lover all his life, and now, when he could hold on to so little of his own recall, he welcomed the chance to have something to call his own.

Well, one day I came in for a visit, and his dog was lying on its side.

My dad was not petting it as usual.

He looked up at me and said, "Did this dog die again?"

My mind froze, literally. He expressed his concern so matter-of-factly that it actually threw me back against the walls of my own reality.

I think I physically staggered a bit.

I wanted to laugh, but I did not.

I saw his face, so sincere, so puzzled and distressed by this possibility. This impossible possibility.

I regained my balance quickly, instinctively, and, like a trapeze artist suspended momentarily in the air, I grabbed for dear life in the direction of my intention for kindness over rightness.

"I think so, Papa," I said. "But not to worry, it's only temporary."

I'm happy to say the wee Yorkie had regained his full sentinel stature by the end of the visit.

What was happening?

Was he like a child who talks to a toy as if it has life because he craved the companionship?

I think sometimes he knew it wasn't alive, but he also knew that he thought it was alive. So he knew something odd was up, and it soothed him to pet that dog as if they were comrades-in-arms, as if they were both being duped.

What's Your Name Again?

Very early on, my dad was aware, if not willing to admit it openly, that something was not as it should be with his recall or recognition of simple processes. Perhaps he actually felt different, or perhaps he could tell by my odd responses to some of his behaviours.

So in order to appear "still in the game," he would constantly play tricks on me about his memory. Apparently, everyone else could tell when he was joshing me, so they got a great kick out of this. He would suddenly say, "What's your name again?" knowing full well what my name was.

At the time, I thought the joker in him enjoyed the momentary fire of panic in my eyes and the thrill of pulling one over on me! Or that he was asking this particular question over and over to keep me wondering if the other lapses in memory were tricks too, so I wouldn't really know what he could or could not remember. It did seem a rather clever way of camouflaging the disability.

My dad had such a bright mind. And as I recalled this behaviour years later, I began to consider another aspect of it altogether. As well as being a trickster, he had also been a consummate teacher to me, even when I was a dull pupil. In light of this then, it is highly probable that, regardless of his failing faculties, he was purposefully trying to prepare me for the day when this might actually happen, when he would no longer recognize me.

I remember well the day it finally did happen.

The day that he didn't recognize me.

It was very close to the end of his battle, and it happened so gently, so easily.

On this day, as I came up to his lunch table, he looked up at me so sweetly and said, "Oh, hi honey, how are you?"

I was ecstatic, because he had been non-verbal for quite a while.

"Oh, hi Papa! It's so good to see you," I chirped, at which point he immediately turned to one of the aides passing by and said, "Oh, hi honey, how are you?" in the very same tone of voice.

It stung for a moment, I will admit, and the nurses and care workers in the room tried to shield me with tender glances.

But he had prepared me well, that beautiful old man. And I found myself feeling grateful instead of hurt. Grateful that I was still one of his "honeys." After all was said and done, that would have to be enough.

And after all was said and done, it was enough . . . thank you, Papa!

Part Two

Dealing with Disorientation

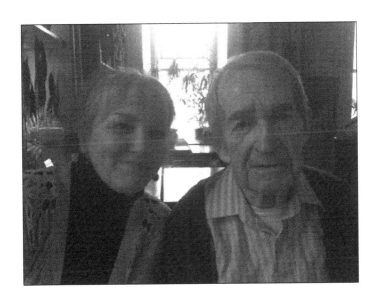

The Glaze over His Eyes

When I first moved into my parents' home, it was primarily to help my mom, who had a number of health issues that required she have assistance with daily activities. We all knew she suspected something odd was up with Dad, but, for the most part, he seemed okay to the rest of the family when we saw him. Cranky as ever, funny as ever, just slower that's all. I knew that taking care of her was not easy for him, so my stay there was meant to be for both their benefit.

And it did seem that he was fine to me, so I could focus mainly on looking after Mom, which I did happily until her death only ten months later.

One day shortly after my mom had passed away, we were preparing to go out for lunch. Dad was getting up from his chair and chatting with my uncle when Makwa pranced into the room. Makwa was my four-year-old dog, who had been close to my dad since he was a pup and barely left his side for fear of losing a cookie opportunity. As he came into the room, my dad exclaimed loudly, "Whose dog is this? What a lovely dog!"

At first, I giggled and searched in his eyes for the proverbial twinkle that always gave my dad away when he was joking. I saw no sign of it. What I saw instead was a glaze over his eyes and that his question was quite sincere. I was completely baffled and then frightened. I remember thinking, "This must be what Mom saw."

Stranger still is the fact that he never again failed to recognize Makwa, who was a faithful companion to him for the next five years. That it happened at all was alarming, though, and it put me on alert, particularly since my dad was still driving to the store each morning to get his paper. I decided to have him seen by a gerontologist to determine if this was an issue that could affect his driving and whether his license should be renewed.

This trip to the doctor's office was my first experience of denial with respect to my dad's increasing memory loss. As we sat in the office, and my dad was given a number of comprehension tests, I coached and prompted him on some of the questions.

By this time, it had become second nature for me to help him with paperwork and such, and, in my mind, I was just lending a hand. When it came to the clock that my dad was asked to draw, I noticed that he left out one of the numbers. Considering it a harmless slip on his part, I pointed out the omission to him, and that was when the doctor politely asked me to stop helping him, because she couldn't make an accurate assessment that way.

I was annoyed at this. I thought, "Well, he knows what a bloody clock is! He's just nervous 'cause it's a test!"

At the time, it was unthinkable that my dad couldn't recognize a clock. He had been fixing watches as a hobby for over 40 years!

In the end, the tests did confirm that there was a developing form of dementia, and my dad's license was suspended.

I felt guilty.

I knew in my heart it was a step we both had to take, but I resisted it almost as much as he did.

Journal Entry: August 19, 2004

Last night I dreamed I came into the kitchen and Mom was making the morning coffee.

She was annoyed at Dad, as per usual, and was struggling to fill a pot at the sink. She bowed her head into the sink, as if weakened by the job and moaned, "He's washing those eggs again."

I looked over to the drying rack to see two piles of dirty eggshells that my dad was washing again.

It was obviously the act of a confused mind. As I turned towards her, she was talking to Dad, who had just walked in the room.

I don't recall what she said, but the tone of her voice was so sincerely kind and compassionate. It surprised me even in my own dream, because her voice was often strained in the last few years with trying to be patient with him.

I was thrilled to see her, even though I thought she had a funny hairdo . . . not like anything I remember her wearing.

I awoke wondering if the dream meant she had

forgiven him for getting dementia.

Journal Entry: February 13, 2005

An odd silence thunders in my head today.

But it isn't really silent, it's kind of hiding quietly.

I think it is fear.

I think I have been hoping my dad's confusion was a temporary something.

Hoping that it would mend somehow, and I could go home.

It's like a secret, a feather falling, a whisper in the night.

I don't want to hear it, so it stays unspoken.

In my mind.

But I know it's there.

Wherever I go.

What will he do if I take way his license?

He will hate me.

Those words paralyze me like never before.

His Disintegration
Struck Bone

When we have to relate constantly with someone with dementia, and with the frayed thought processes that go with this mental disorder, our minds clamour to maintain a sense of order. It can so easily become an irritation to try to follow the splintering that results from flitting from one time frame to another, one reality to another, or one fractured memory to another.

For a professional caregiver who is not as emotionally attached as a family member, this is a learned skill and can be delivered with simplicity and understanding. How very different for a family member, however, and especially a son or daughter. There is a deep history in the psyche, as well as in the emotions, of a relationship that was ordered and functional at one time. So it becomes a matter of learning to respond in a new way as well as cope with the unintentional resistance from the old pattern. Likewise, a spousal caregiver is challenged when an established relationship of trust and dependence is torn from its roots. And a spouse is often elderly and in need of some health or domestic assistance as well. Fortunately, I did have the vitality of relative youth on my side when it came to the stamina needed to keep a constant vigil over my dad's every need. What differed from being a spouse, however, was the fact that he had been in my life since the beginning of it.

I had never known life without my dad and his central role in it. Even though I had gone off and married and raised a family of my own for 30 years, the very roots of my self-image as a child were inextricably intertwined with his. The patterns of mutual expectations and behaviours were well established between us. And so, his mental collapse was something I could not always keep an impartial distance from.

His disintegration struck bone deep and became my own undoing in unexpected ways.

It probably didn't help that the house itself was disintegrating at the same time, and this was a constant source of irritation to me.

My dad wasn't exactly a hoarder, but a pack rat? Oh my, yes.

The house had always been a source of contention for my mom as well, because Dad liked to start handyman projects, but he very rarely finished them. And being a tight-fisted sort, he refused to pay anyone else to do anything he could potentially do.

When I came to live there, the basement looked like a collector's heaven, with paperback books by the hundreds lining what narrow passageway remained to get to the washing machine. His tool area, which had once been organized in impressive little cubbies, had exploded into an anarchy of nails, and screws, and stuff I didn't recognize. The rec room was just a sad old tribute to the past, and its best-before date for health reasons alone had long expired.

Any attempt I made to upgrade or improve the condition of the basement actually enraged my dad, because, in his mind, I was interfering without permission with his man cave and his future projects.

The garage was no better, though, admittedly, much of the clutter in there was storage from my own dismantled house.

As his dementia advanced, his inability to let go of control also advanced.

But so did mine.

There were times when I myself became so frustrated at his

stubborn refusal to let me improve the condition of our home, to bring some order to the chaos, that I reverted to petulant behaviours, too . . . at which point we would both stomp through the house pouting, even snarling, or giving each other the cold shoulder.

It sounds comical describing it now, but it was far from funny at the time.

Journal Entry: October 20, 2004

This assignment is too much for me, and I need to pray for deliverance.

This is difficult to do, because I assume deliverance means something I also don't want to think about . . .

I know he wouldn't do well in a home.

He'd feel abandoned like when he was a child.

I just cannot do that to him!

But I recognize the signs of my own crumbling, and I know I cannot hold up much longer in this situation.

It is very sad to have to admit this.

I think it might be different; I might have the strength, if we were living in my home closer to my friends and family. I am pretty much captive here in his home with no friends nearby.

I find it an unreasonable situation for anyone to have to endure, and I am no martyr. Yet, and yet, I love my dad.

So I am conflicted, as well as trapped—in this

house; mentally, by his illness that is so persistently exhausting; and emotionally, because I love him as well, and I want him taken care of as much as I want some breathing space of my own.

Dad is growing more befuddled about everything.

Sadly, I know just how that feels.

Journal Entry: December 1, 2004

I guess we've been in a hiatus for a week or so.

The issue of the car has receded to a common ache—a dull roar.

Ron (my brother), has been staying here for two weeks now, and, each evening when he comes after work, Dad asks him why he's here.

I wonder why he keeps forgetting that he said Ron could stay here for a while.

He acts like he is king of the castle, defending it from a rogue prince.

Maybe he really thinks that.

He is becoming increasingly irritable, and, today, I may just stay out of his way.

Sue is here, so I can go out somewhere for an hour.

He probably needs a break from me too.

He is also becoming very vocal about wanting to save his money. "No Christmas lights" is one example—it is making me dizzy.

One minute he is someone I love and respect and

the next minute someone I don't like at all.

This is going to be one helluvaday.

It is pouring outside, so he can't even escape to go for a walk.

It must be so confusing and disturbing to him to be losing his freedom on the heels of losing Mom.

I have been trying to save him from his own feelings, a habit I picked up many years ago as a child.

Now I don't want to save my father from his own feelings, partly because they are irrational and mean-spirited, and I don't want anything to do with them.

But the other point is that it is probably time that I let that habit go altogether.

They are not my feelings.

What are my feelings? That is what I am left with.

Journal Entry: January 11, 2005

I think I write each morning to try to establish a reality for myself that is not driven by my dad's energy or perspective.

Something like a soothing blanket to draw around myself for protection or maybe even camouflage.

But I feel guilty that I stay here and still wish I was somewhere else.

It's like walking around in two pieces, in opposite directions.

I wonder if poor Dad feels like this, too.

I need to make some sense of this for myself so that I do not succumb to this feeling of fissure and crack up myself.

My dad is so vulnerable sometimes, so infuriating at others.

I think that when Dad drops in his own capabilities I drop in mine.

He has stopped setting the table for breakfast more often now.

This morning, he just sat at a messy table and read the paper until I got up to set it and make him something to eat.

I feel like he is giving up, and it makes me mad.

I can't give up now, can I?

My heart has no end of patience for him, but my mind is a raging bull.

And God knows Dad taught me well how to act like one.

Alzheimer's Voice

Then, there is the story within the story that cannot be given words.

That which actually refuses to come forward.

That which my sense of protection still will not allow me to divulge about my dad.

Anyone who has or is now caring for a loved one with Alzheimer's knows exactly what I am referring to. There are nightmare situations that are simply too raw to talk about.

Let's be honest. There is a degree of shame around some Alzheimer's behaviours, especially the ones that are so far removed from the lifelong personalities.

For some caregivers it definitely becomes abusive during the "sundowning" period. Describing the details of abuse can be rife with disbelief and shame, and the response of the family caregiver may mirror the response of other domestic abuse sufferers. Silence.

Often family members outside the household itself don't even know what is happening, because of this secrecy.

My brother Ron knew the barrage of verbal abuse that I had to bear from our dad.

He knew Dad couldn't help it.

I knew Dad couldn't help it.

More often than not, Dad had no idea what he was doing let alone that he couldn't help it.

And even with the supportive family that we had, there were a few close members who refused to believe what was happening behind closed doors and made me the brunt of their criticism.

They chose to disbelieve because it was easier than facing the facts, just as they chose to criticize to mask their own guilt for not helping more.

Complex? Tricky? Confusing? Oh my, yes.

It did seem that being around the house was an instant source of exaggerated misery and negative behaviour for my dad. As I look back now, it is so clear. My mom was simply not there, and as much as we tried to muddle on together, the loneliness and fury over her loss was a thorn in his soul that never went away.

One of the marital patterns of coping with stress or disagreeable issues that had existed openly between my parents was my dad's fondness for escaping by leaving the house in his car.

No one ever asked where he went, and he didn't stay away too long.

He just escaped.

I think this made the removal of his car keys and the inability to escape unwelcome encounters with me harder than one would expect. And it triggered his rage.

Frankie's voice: "I'll just go for a quick drive and let the air clear."

Alzheimer's voice: "Where are my keys you stupid bitch?"

Daughter's voice: "Dad, you are not allowed to drive anymore, remember?"

Alzheimer's voice: "Liar!"

Journal Entry: December 7, 2004

Dear God, every day I ask for the same thing.

Peace.

Peace in my heart.

Peace of mind.

World peace.

Peace in my life.

Peace in my children's lives.

And every day (well most), I wake up feeling agitated and completely peaceless and work toward my desire for Peace as the day wears on.

I wake up weary.

I wake up tired.

I wake up feeling defeated.

His confusion and suspicious mind drive me easily from the centre of my own peace.

I need prayers to remind me to return to the eye.

While he storms around the house.

Furious in his grief.

Furious that he is losing control.

Every day I ask for the same thing along with

peace.

I ask for escape from this burden.

And yet I love my dad.

And I am committed to doing the right thing by my mom in caring for him.

And it is a burden still.

So in my own conflict I look, I search, I desire, I beg for peace.

This is my conflict.

Raging away in my soul.

Alzheimer's Takes No Prisoners

I don't think I have ever met a person as socially friendly as my dad was.

I often called him a chick magnet, and, though he did have a fondness for making the girls smile, he was happy to engage men and women alike in friendly chit-chat whenever he could. A curious character trait, since, as I have already mentioned, he fought anyone and everyone anytime he could as a young man. I never asked him when it all changed. I just knew that somewhere along the line he outgrew the need to punch his way through life.

No doubt the war had a sobering effect on him as it did on his entire generation, and he landed on his feet after it was over, with a different appreciation for his fellow man.

So too, a forty-year career as an industrial methods analyst encouraged this amiable side of his nature. His job, as I recall, was to stroll around the factory floor all day long chatting with the machinists and assembly workers, in order to analyze the workflow for efficiency.

He carried this well-worn behaviour into his private life as well. When we went camping in the summers, it was not uncommon for him to disappear for hours during a five-minute walk to the water pump. He would stop at every campsite along the way to chat with the campers. I mean *every* campsite. By the time we had finished our vacation, my dad knew most of the people in the park. I knew this, because they would all stop to say goodbye to him as they were breaking camp and leaving.

Later, after he retired, it was the neighbours on the street that were the lucky recipients of his door-to-door congeniality. Then, even after his initial diagnosis of Alzheimer's, when he and I went out for dinner, he would stop at as many tables on the way to the door as he could, always with a little quip, sure to bring a laugh to the other patrons.

It was one of his most endearing characteristics, and, even now, it is painful to consider how the eventual isolation he felt because of this merciless illness robbed him of this simple and generous pleasure.

Alzheimer's takes no prisoners. It broke my dad's mind and it broke my heart.

Journal Entry: December 16, 2004

BROKEN

One of my wings is broken so I won't fly away, I

guess

So I'll stay in the coop.

Sad little songbird

Tending a broken wing in a broken nest

With a broken heart

And a broken little Papa Snowbird.

Perched on the couch my soul calls out the window

A muffled one-note song

Broken, broken, broken

To no one in the trees

They are all bare—

All gone south

To escape the cold and ice

And pain.

Best to Let It Be

My ambition for my Dad was to make everything all right by trying to neutralize, or at least minimize, the theft of Alzheimer's. I didn't think I was in denial per se, I just wanted to keep him as present and aware of himself as I could, by gently reminding him about his life and the "who's who" in it. I guess I was trying to coax his awareness into recall.

I felt it was a viable way of helping him preserve his dignity, but I see now it was, in large part, for me and my concept of his dignity.

It was only in the last year, the year he fell so far into the abyss of fractured recall that I relinquished my quest in this and let him say and be whatever the moment demanded.

As I look back, armed with what I know now about Alzheimer's, I feel a certain amount of remorse for the way I pushed him to be his best for so long. I suppose I was only following what I had learned from him as a child. He had never allowed me to be satisfied with my own second best, and so I had excelled at nearly everything I tried. I also wonder now if it wasn't selfishly driven by my need for his company as I tried to be my best and stay propped up for the challenges that came each day.

Near the end, when his best was so fragile and hazy, my best was to summon a smile when I came to visit and say, "Hey, handsome, how's it going today?"

From there, we both just did the best we could with what we had.

Journal Entry: August 11, 2011

It's getting harder to take Papa out for lunch now.

Even harder to watch his enthusiasm for going out take such a downturn.

It's almost like I am the one who needs to keep this habit going, not him.

He is content to sit in his room and look out the window.

I miss our walks.

I miss our talks.

Oh well, chocolate doughnuts are what binds us now, not too shabby. I guess.

Part Three

Moving Past the Battle

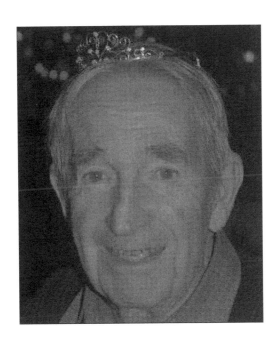

No Longer in the Driver's Seat

Dad wasn't ready, willing, or able to relinquish his licence.

He had been driving for over 70 years. He had driven to Florida and back once a year for over 20 years.

He had taught me the art of defensive driving long before it was even a concept in the driver education programs.

He had been an exemplary driver all his life, and he still felt that way, saw himself that way.

No uppity doctor or government ministry was going to take that away from him. Oh no.

So guess who was left with the task?

I felt bad about this, I really did, but the anxiety over what skill or road rule would suddenly fail him while he was driving to the store for his morning paper was getting unbearable.

We lived in a neighbourhood loaded with little kids and with a fire hall just down the street. What else could I do?

Since his car was still in the garage, and he still had his own keys, I tried to explain as gently as I could what the situation was and why he couldn't drive anymore.

One day he would understand and not go out for the paper, and the next he'd be out the door and down the street before I could stop him. Neighbours would call to let me know he was "on the loose."

At first, I tried to remove his keys from the key hook, but he was wise to me, and it not only infuriated him but also hurt his feelings. He told me he felt as if I didn't trust his ability to honour his promise not to drive. Unfortunately, he was not aware that his mind was shifting from day to day, so trust was not the issue.

Journal Entry: November 16, 2004

The official notice of Dad's suspension came yesterday. Even though he has only a week to wait to see his doctor for a possible letter of reinstatement, he went for a paper this morning all huffy and angry and belligerent. He is forcing me to take his keys, because he refuses to act responsibly.

It will be ugly, I suppose.

He will be ugly, I suppose.

He will have a tantrum, so I must decide where I want to be when it happens. I could phone the police and report his behaviour—let them come and impound his car. How harsh does this lesson have to be? Why?

His belligerence is toxic and abusive. The harshness is his creation, not mine.

Impounding his car seems to be the only way to stop him from driving. Or I could just go out and take the damn garage door opener.

Or I could try slamming doors and cursing every other second word—all the techniques he seems to admire for causing such discomfort that he gets his own way.

I am furious inside right now. Why should I let a feeble-minded, stubborn old man continue to create such a bad atmosphere?

So I'll remove myself today. He can stew all he wants.

He shuffles around the kitchen, cursing away, but he's deaf enough that he mutters under his breath like a fool. It might even be sad to an onlooker, but to me it is infuriating.

Journal Entry: November 17, 2004

Dad has left the house—without his cane.

He is furious.

His car wouldn't start this morning, because the lights had been left on all night. By yours truly, of course.

He asked to borrow my car, and when I reminded him that he doesn't have a valid driver's licence, he got very angry.

It is too bad, because this is the first time he has asked to borrow my car, and it must have been hard for him to do even that.

And I said, "No."

I don't know where he has gone.

I do know he feels terribly alone right now.

It is so sad.

He has a sense that this is a trick to get him to stop driving.

Where has he gone?

Journal Entry: November 22, 2004

Don't exactly know what my dad is going through.

I didn't take his keys or his door opener this morning.

Something told me to let him alone today—to let him make the decision, one way or the other, to drive or not to drive.

I expected to hear him slip out quietly this morning to drive over to get a paper. Instead, he did the dishes first thing, so I had to get up.

Now he is in his bedroom quietly doing something. Maybe preparing to go outside—really, I sense he is struggling because he knows he told me he wouldn't drive, and now he has to keep his word or break it.

Funny the things he does remember.

But it has become important for him to come to the decision himself.

He has put his coat on, and if he drives it will be his decision, not mine.

He has donned his coat as I write and is going

for a paper.

Will he walk or drive? God bless his heart, he just walked past the window.

I am so glad I followed the prompting to "let go and let God."

My dad did the good thing.

He kept his word to me.

He chose to walk.

Oops—now he is back.

I think he is getting the car.

Oh, well. He is struggling, I know.

Funny, he would go about it this way.

It's as if I am being asked to disable the car.

Okay—that was a plan anyway.

God keep him and everyone else out of harm's way until he returns.

Helen (the neighbourhood watch-guard) just called to let me know he has taken the car.

It will be interesting to see what happens today.

I will not address it directly at all.

I will pretend I don't even know.

He needs to stew in his own sneaky juices—or

maybe not.

I hope he enjoys the trip, because it will be the last one he ever takes in the driver's seat. So let it be surrounded in peace, God.

He deserves that.

It looks like a great day for a walk in the woods.

Hijacking the Car

After a few weeks of circling around the futile pattern of divesting Dad of his car keys only to have him demand them back, my brother and I felt it was time to devise a plan or two.

Plan one had been simply to hide the garage door opener. It had an annoying habit of being lost or misplaced anyway, so it seemed to be a reasonable ruse. It was only meant to be a temporary measure, though, since my dad had stuff in the garage that he liked to tinker with, and I didn't want to shrink his world even more.

The tricky part of all this was the unpredictability of Dad's condition as well as the extreme mood swings his mental deterioration caused. One day I could keep him safe with the slightest deception, and wham, the next day he was all over the situation like a sleuth.

So Operation Garage Door Opener didn't last but a few days when plan two—hijacking the car—sprang into action. This plan involved disabling the car itself so that it simply could not be driven.

Two tires went mysteriously flat overnight.

It is sad to admit that this worked at first because my dad would forget from day to day that it had happened, and yet it is sadder to admit that I had to tell barefaced lies to him to make it work. Even now, I feel a tinge of remorse over my role in this scheme, but short of taking his car away like he was a child, we saw no other way to achieve the goal while keeping him involved in the process.

When this plan, too, became a source of suspicion to him, we charged for the finish line, went for the gusto, and shamelessly deadened the battery.

Then, after a few days of recharging the battery and trips to the gas station to fill the tires, my dad declared one day that he wanted to sell "the piece of shit."

I was relieved.

We were both tired of the daily ordeal, and I was doing the worst thing possible—I was numbing out. I was numbing out because constantly lying to my dad was deeply offensive to me, and it left me feeling ashamed, defective, helpless . . . ironically the very feelings I was trying to save him from feeling through this difficult passage.

Journal Entry: November 19, 2004

Last night, Dad announced that he wants to sell his car. The tire has gone mysteriously flat and the battery is dead too.

It's too much for him to handle, so he wants to let go of the whole affair.

I hope he stays on this track.

He seems to (well, last night he did) enjoy the feeling of making the decision himself and being in the driver's seat, so to speak, over how it will all go down.

I'm glad.

However, I realize that it could all revert today.

He is fairly unstable these days.

I just move one day at a time.

At least today he wore a coat to go and get the paper, and his dog is on a leash.

He is reinventing his own routine, and for my dad at 85, that is a miracle, truly!

He has just returned from walking to get the paper and is on a rant about his licence.

So I'm not sure where the idea of selling his car
has gone.

I am prepared to just remove the keys from the
house.

Having the car fixed is a first step anyway.

He may have to take a few runs at this.

That's okay. I'll hold his hand as he tries.

Journal Entry: November 21, 2004

So here's the circle we are rolling around, I guess.

For two days, Dad talked about selling his car.

He asked me to jump-start the car and inflate the tires so we could put it on the market.

I did those things.

Then he asked me if we could drive it to The Bluffs instead of my car, just to keep it in good shape.

We did that (I drove, of course).

Then Saturday came along, and as he was making his breakfast he angrily announced that he was not selling his car.

I had to go to work for a few hours, so I lifted his keys from the holder.

As I was going out the door, he confronted me about the keys—so he obviously was watching those keys very carefully.

He ordered me to put them back, which I refused to do, and we had an unpleasant altercation.

I called him from my cell, on my way to work, to apologize.

He said it's as if I don't trust him and that he isn't going to drive anyway.

I felt terrible and told him that it isn't him I don't trust—it is his ability to remember not to drive.

So this morning when I awoke, his keys had been removed from the holder. He was very quick to wake up and snatch them.

Why does he need them?

I am going to remove the garage door opener again—so I guess we are back at square one.

I know he wants to go for a beer today. Maybe he will ask to be taken.

I have to admit, I am expecting a fight again.

This is strangely exhausting.

I think the battery needs to go dead again.

Journal Entry: December 3, 2004

And so we begin a new relationship.

My dad has his feelings. I have mine.

He arose today and went out to get a paper.

He stopped by the car on the way and came back into the house. "Piece of shit!" he said. I guess that's the car he's talking about.

I guess it wouldn't start again.

I guess he forgot we removed the battery, and it's in my back seat.

Oh well.

Then he set out boldly to get a paper.

Didn't go far—I guess it's cold outside.

I got dressed and ready to be asked for help, but he's not talking to me—no "Good morning."

Nothing.

I guess I'm the piece of shit.

Those appear to be his feelings.

Here are mine:

I am completely willing to help him when he asks.

I know it is hard, even excruciating for him to ask for help. Probably where I learned the same selfish behaviour.

Perhaps it is the thing he has come to learn before he passes.

To ask for help.

I sense that he doesn't want to be beholden to anyone by asking for help.

It means for him that he would be vulnerable to being used or abused.

Or like me, he sees it as a sign of weakness, a weakness that becomes public with the asking.

A weakness that invites ridicule and shame.

So I will not jump in every time I see him struggling.

He'd rather suffer in silence than ask me to go for a paper.

He's silently having breakfast and reading a flyer.

Perhaps he is waiting for me to offer.

When I did offer to go the other day, he said, "Suit yourself."

So difficult for him to express gratitude.

It must be uncomfortable for him to feel it.

Those are his feelings.

My feelings? To let him be.

He is creating the silence and distance between us today, so let him.

The Happy Finish Line

After my mom had passed, with my dad's blessing I made the decision to ask their longtime housekeeper Susan if she would stay on.

I didn't need the help with housework, but she had become a faithful friend to my parents over the years, and I knew my dad needed the reassurance of her presence to bridge the gap my mom's absence had created. She also had become my friend and served as a willing respite for me once a week.

When she heard that Dad was thinking of selling his car, she asked me discreetly if I thought he would consider selling it to her. Her own car had recently broken down completely, so

I didn't hesitate in putting the question to him, and he seemed quite pleased with the idea.

It's practical wisdom that it's not wise to sell a previously owned car to a family member or close friend. I think it is because the unforeseen problems that inevitably arise with a used vehicle can inadvertently cause hard feelings. My brother and I discussed the potential sale from this, as well as other points of view, but in the end it was my dad who made the final decision to say yes to her.

I think it made him feel good to help her out.

I think it made him feel less stranded to know that his car was going to someone close by, someone he knew would appreciate it.

I also think he enjoyed the idea of being able to keep an eye on it, once a week, when she came to visit.

In the end, it turned out to be a win-win for all of us.

He sold it for a fair price to her and she took great care of it for him.

This transaction settled his soul regarding the whole licence/driving affair, and, from that day forward, he was happy to have me chauffeur him everywhere.

Hallelujah, he was happy.

I was happy.

My dad had turned me into a Trekkie years earlier so one

could say . . .

My prime directive was accomplished!

Like the Three Stooges in a Fix

One of my main concerns as my dad's comprehension of his world and how to behave in it crumbled was to make sure that his dignity was protected. And, with what I considered all good intention, I was fierce in this quest.

One day, Dad and I were out for lunch with my brother, Ron, and the conversation turned, as it so often did, to the glasses he was wearing. His eyesight had been declining, and I had been trying to keep his prescription up-to-date with the changes.

So on this particular day, he was declaring rather assertively that the glasses on the table beside his plate, the same glasses he had just taken off his face, were, in fact, not his glasses! As far as he was concerned, they never had been his glasses and never could be his glasses, because they simply did not work! His language was pretty colourful, and he was certain that someone was pulling a fast one on him with a foreign pair of glasses.

"Dad," I said, "I assure you these are your glasses, but they just need to be upgraded. Don't wear them if they bother you. We'll get it sorted out in a few days."

Lunch continued on, but each time he saw the glasses beside his plate the same conversation sparked up, and he became increasingly agitated. Finally, Ron said, "Dad, just put the glasses away in your pocket for now."

So my Dad picked up what he thought were the glasses and, with a panache to rival Clark Gable, elegantly slipped them into his shirt pocket.

What he didn't realize was that he had plucked a chewed chicken bone from his lunch plate instead of his glasses.

Now, I had seen my dad tuck his glasses into his shirt pocket hundreds of times over the years, always with this same flair, this same bold certainty.

Suddenly I didn't know what to do or where to look.

In my eyes, he looked so silly, so undignified, and so vulnerable to humiliation. And what did my brother do? He doubled over laughing like a damned hyena!

There we were, like the Three Stooges in a fix—my dad innocently chewing on his lunch with a bare chicken bone sticking out of his breast pocket, my brother choking in hysterics behind his menu, and me, fuming like a dragon at the whole dangerous affair.

I was angry because I felt my brother's laughter was insensitive and made Dad the brunt of a joke, robbing him of his rightful dignity. However, in a recent conversation with a good friend, as we were recalling this story, she said quite matter-of-factly, "Well, you know, your dad would have found that very funny, too, if he had been able."

Her innocent words had a strange effect on me. I found myself being instantly transported in a kind of daydream back in time, back to that very day.

There I saw my dad, chicken bone and all, blissfully enjoying his lunch, satisfied that the blasted conversation about the glasses had been resolved. And there was my brother, with whom I had been angry enough to kick several times under the table, laughing away, unable to control himself.

This time, I saw it differently.

This time, I saw that my brother was laughing partly for himself and partly for our dad. And I saw that he knew, from years of experience with this man, something I was not privy to. He knew from their countless adventures in fishing huts, around card tables, and other places that only the "boys" went, that it was not just funny, but a kind of funny our dad loved.

I saw that my brother was actually laughing for him, not at him.

"It's just not right," I remember saying over and over about that laughter.

Now here, all these years later, in an unexpected gift of insight, I realized that, caught up as I had been in my demand for dignity, I had failed to recognize an instinctive kindness and respect my brother was showing to our father.

Still to this day, my brother chuckles like a kid when we recall this memory and insists, "It was funny!"

But I don't kick him any more.

Journal Entry: December 9, 2004

With each new thing that disappears and each new time my dad accuses me of stealing, I lose a bit of my confidence and grip on what I thought I could do here to help him.

I can't keep looking for my chequebook, the car papers, Rachel's necklace, my engagement ring etc., etc.!

I know he saw it on my dresser and thought it was Mom's.

I know he can't help what he's doing.

Now my purse is missing!

What, do I have to lock my room every time I leave it?

Am I in prison here? I want to fall down and cry, and I dreamed last night I started smoking again.

What's happening to me?

I've always been so strong.

Ron tells me to lighten up, that it's funny, in a way.

Not when it happens every day!

It's a Family Affair

It is commonly acknowledged in the field of therapy and counselling that any form of mental illness, including addiction, is a family experience.

The effects of the affliction are not confined to one person's experience.

Alzheimer's is no different.

In spite of the diverse responses that family members may have to this terrible condition, everyone is affected in some way.

More often than not, adversely.

Even those who tune out, turn off, and drop out are likely doing so because of denial or guilt or shame or the biggest one—

fear. Often, family members may appear to have no feelings about it in order to cope. Unfortunately, this makes them less apt to visit or support those who are actively involved in the care.

I was blessed with a wonderful support group of friends and family for the most part. However, my decision to move my dad from his home after living with him there for four years was met with a barrage of criticism and hurtful accusations.

I knew that these responses were fear-, and anger-, and in some cases guilt-based and not intentionally meant as personal attacks. Still, they were personal, and it was tremendously difficult to bear the brunt of these emotions from those I had thought of as close allies—especially when I was already so frail and vulnerable from the years spent with my dad.

I have only one brother, so the common problem of dissention among siblings over the how/when/where of this process did not exist. Ron's support and encouragement throughout the entire time with our dad was remarkable.

He was my pillar.

He openly acknowledged that he simply could not do what I was doing. He could not deal emotionally with Dad's decline day to day, and yet he was there to listen and sympathize with every crisis call I placed to him.

He once told me that he had always admired the way I stood up to Dad as a teenager when I believed there was a cause to. He said that he could never do that, and he considered it a strength I possessed . . . a strength that I also brought to the mission of caring for Dad when he was not able to care for himself.

Strangely enough, I remember my teenage years as rebellious and somewhat disrespectful, but Ron was right about one thing. I did bring that same feisty attitude to the table years later when Alzheimer's came to dinner . . . I stood up to it; I fought back; I argued, and I would not back down!

Everyone in the family was freaked out after the Big Mistake on July 11 (in Part Four) when I moved my dad away from the old family homestead and closer to where I needed to live with my family and friends. Hell, the old neighbourhood had changed drastically anyway, and there were only one or two of the original folks left there.

What was the problem?

Change.

That's what the problem was. Change and the fear of it.

One of my sons was upset with me for doing this to his "Baba" as he was called by my children. He felt that his Baba should be allowed to stay in his home and die there as he wanted to. But to me that meant finding him at the foot of the stairs because of a fall, or hearing that he was hit by a car running after his dog, or risking him setting the house on fire somehow.

I argued that I simply couldn't do that, and I meant no disrespect to Baba's wishes to stay in his home. I explained that my sole concern and duty, as I saw it, was to keep Baba safe. Still, it was an issue between us for quite some time. And then . . . and then . . . in the last two days of my dad's life who was there keeping vigil with me beside his bed? That same son, with that same huge love for his Baba regardless of our past disagreement.

Ron's kids were afraid for their "Grampa" (as they called him) as well and buckled at the thought of losing their own ties to the home they had known since they were born.

We all grieved in our own way at this particular rite of passage for my dad, and, in hindsight, I can fully understand the gut twists and turns it unintentionally caused.

The family flailing continued for the next year until my dad actually moved into a nursing home, and the kids settled into visiting when they could.

Journal Entry: March 20, 2007

No, no, no, I am not doing well here at all.

It feels like there is a kind of dark mood settled across my shoulders like a death shawl.

I have the sense that if I just don't move it will go away.

Slip off as quickly as it appeared and slither away like a receding shadow.

I wish it was a cloak of invisibility instead of a cloak of despair.

My family have run away in fear.

I didn't see that coming, but I should have.

But where the hell did they all go?

I can't run away.

I won't run away.

Some things hit you from behind and bring you to your knees.

From the Shadows

My dad had developed a curious habit of whistling to himself, quietly, just under his breath. He usually did it when he was puttering or wandering around the house, and I knew where he was by this sound.

Whistling was far more common years ago than it is now, and whistling quietly in this manner was not unusual for gentleman of his generation. It was an endearing sound and usually indicated to me that he was in a good frame of mind, even if he was looking for, as he would say, "Something fishy going on here."

I remember thinking at the time that it probably gave him

something constant to tether his attention to.

But now as I review so much more of his life and see him in this expanded context, I am compelled to consider yet another intention he might have had for this habit. I think Alzheimer's was like a suspicious companion that taunted him from the shadows. So perhaps his whistling was like the whistling one might do in an unfamiliar dark alley to prove you're not afraid— a way to communicate your nonchalant bravery to whoever might be lurking in the shadows.

Journal Entry: November 22, 2004

SHADOW BOXER

See the lonely figure
Spinning and prancing around the ring,
Circling the elusive foe—
The one he casts before himself
To keep the action alive.

No one blows the whistle on this champion's game
Without his permission.
Like cunning footwork,
His breathing whistles a distraction to the oppo-
nent,
Hypnotizing the light to expose the spy—
The suspicious companion that is al-
ways there, taunting him.

His blood flows in my veins
Like rapids over worn-down things.
I recognize the swings the shadow boxer throws.
From my ringside seat.

Alzheimer's Oasis

As my dad's full-time caregiver, I was impelled to follow a routine each day that was generated by his level of abilities. I found that his capacity to function and be content was directly related to the predictability of our daily activities. Any divergence from a strict pattern was quite upsetting to him. He relied on the simple routine of everyday sameness to keep him feeling safe and coherent. I think it was like his whistling really; it assuaged the tremendous fear of mental anarchy that hid in the shadows and constantly threatened him.

There were three routines that kept my dad free from agitation and behaving pleasantly. We engaged in these activities almost every day, and I enjoyed this time with him very much.

Happy Hour

My dad liked his martinis with a twist of lemon and exactly two drops of vermouth.

My dad liked Happy Hour.

He was not, nor had he ever been, a heavy drinker, and I had never once in my life seen him drunk or out of control over alcohol. But he insisted on Happy Hour. He would make one martini only. And then later, when he grew confused over the details of making this revered cocktail, I took over as barmaid and made him a martini with a twist every day at 4:00 p.m.

It was an undisputed ritual.

I, myself, didn't drink gin, couldn't even handle the smell . . . but I easily made an exception for Frankie's martini at Happy Hour.

He had been celebrating Happy Hour for well over 30 years since his retirement, regardless of whatever else may have been going on in his life. More importantly, he had been spending Happy Hour with my mom every day of that 30 years!

It had its own special energy, Happy Hour did. It was like a bubble where time itself stopped, the phone was allowed to go unanswered, and even the dogs knew not to fuss or whine.

It was the most peaceful hour of the day.

As I look back now, I recognize that there was something almost meditative or sacred about it. In the winter, we would watch shows on the TV, but in the warmer weather we would sit on the patio and just listen to the sweet sounds of nature.

We never discussed anything controversial or unpleasant at Happy Hour. It was strictly *verboten*. Even the rules of Happy Hour were never discussed.

I guess it was like high tea to us, because along with the ritual of it all, it carried a certain elegance. My dad would often change his shirt for Happy Hour, and I would refresh my lipstick.

Even if my Dad and I were having a bad day from his behaviours or my impatience, even if we arrived at 4:00 p.m. scratched and frayed, Happy Hour saved the day by delivering a cease-fire zone for us both to recoup, relax, and re-engage.

Happy Hour was far more important than I ever realized at the time.

Solvitur Ambulando

"It is solved by walking."
—St. Augustine

We walked every day.
Even in the winter.

Unless it was too icy for safety's sake.

We walked because the dogs needed the exercise.

We walked because we both needed to get out of the house and feel open space between us and around us.

We walked because it was so enjoyable to be in the peace and quiet of the woods, or the field, or the park, or anywhere we could let the dogs loose to romp and roam freely.

We had at least five favourite places that we walked in, some close by to the house and some that required a drive in the country to reach, and we were free to choose which one matched the whim of the day.

Sometimes we talked and sometimes we just walked in silence.

Like Happy Hour, it was never forced.

It was like a walking meditation, really, much the way labyrinths are.

Our walks often reminded me of labyrinth walking when we would meander in a circle along the path, and double back to where the car was parked.

We both emerged from those walks refreshed and peaceful.

The dogs loved these walks, too.

My dad loved the dogs.

I loved the woods.

It was a win-win-win all 'round.

I miss those walks terribly.

The Pub-Crawl

One of my dad's favourite pleasures was to go out for lunch or dinner. And so we did, every day without fail for five years, with the sole exception of family gatherings and holidays.

It was either lunch or dinner, and sometimes it was both.

This was not because I couldn't or wouldn't cook, and, indeed, it was an expenditure that added up. But it was an activity that made Dad happy, and my brother and I decided that though it seemed an extravagance to us, it was, after all, his money to spend as he wished.

He recognized the ritual of restaurant etiquette, and he so enjoyed kibitzing with the "girl" who regularly served us.

We had at least one preferred restaurant, most often a pub, in each area where we walked the dogs. This included cottage country as well, when we went to visit my brother for a few days.

Frankie was so charming when he was out in public. Nothing about being in a social setting triggered any of his aggressive behaviours. In fact, he was in his element with the undivided attention of the servers. He clearly held centre stage, and he rose with great humour and gusto to the occasion very time.

The waitresses, as I mentioned, loved his entertaining antics, and many became very fond of our dinner visits. Some would literally cheer as we strolled through the front door!

I was just the sideman at these appearances—like Barney to Fred in *The Flintstones.* He was definitely the main attraction at every meal!

One Last Breath

My dad took his last breath on Christmas Eve, 2012 at 8:00 p.m.

Anyone who has been present for the moment of passing of a loved one never forgets the experience. In every detail, it is a remarkable and sacred moment; a phenomenon we neither fully understand nor fully accept. It seems that the grieving process that follows gives us a chance to catch up with the mysterious finality of that moment.

Even though my dad had been disappearing for some time, and quite dramatically in the last year, that final breath of his life was no less profound for me.

During his last few days, I was able to stay camped in his room with the kind permission of the nurses and caregivers at the home. Because it was the Christmas season, I set up a table with sweets and other goodies for whoever might come by to pay their last respects to him, before leaving for the holidays.

He was in a very deep sleep at this point and not in any discomfort, due in part to the informed and compassionate intervention of my daughter-in-law Rachel who was a palliative nurse by profession.

The atmosphere was gentle and quiet as soft Christmas music wafted across the room.

My son, Oadi, (his eldest grandson) had been there all day to keep vigil with me, and, by the evening, my niece Melody (his eldest granddaughter) had come as well. She brought the wake, in the form of three martinis . . . one for her, one for me, and one for "Frankie"!

He couldn't drink it, of course, but that was not the point.

And in keeping with the magical feel of the event, Sare, a young friend of the family made a surprise visit to see him and wish him Godspeed. She had grown close to Frankie in the previous few years as one of his caregivers and had shared many a gin martini with him at family gatherings. Silently he passed the torch to her, and she accepted the honour.

We passed the early evening telling stories, welcoming staff and family visitors, and toasting his life with our martinis. The stories we shared ran the gamut from spiritual philosophy to ghostly encounters to our favourite Frankie adventures.

It was not sad, and it was not solemn, and we laughed a lot during that vigil.

Then at 8:00 p.m., in the middle of one of our Christmas Eve toasts, I heard his breathing change.

I went to hold him and saw him breathe his last.

That was it.

No loud fanfare.

No unearthly clamour of trumpets.

Just silence.

Later that evening, as I sat pondering that moment, I did some computations in my mind to try to grasp the sheer scope of it all.

He breathed one more time and then just stopped.

I estimated that in his lifetime he had breathed one breath every six seconds.

10 breaths every minute,

600 breaths every hour,

14,400 breaths every day,

100,800 breaths every week,

5,241,600 breaths every year.

And then suddenly, when he just didn't take one more

breath at 93 years of age, he had breathed 487,468,800 times!

How could this be?

Why breathe that many times just to suddenly not do it any longer?

That many times!

To me, it was as unfathomable as the stars in the sky, and as vastly overwhelming that after four hundred and eighty-seven million, four hundred and sixty-eight thousand, and eight hundred breaths, he just stopped.

One last quiet breath.

And it was the most piercing sound imaginable.

Part Four

The Ups and Downs of Finding Help

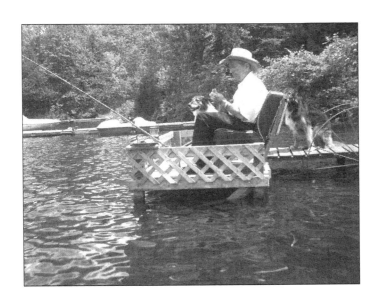

The Big Mistake on July 11th

Moving into a home away from home can be a difficult transition for any senior, even if dementia is not a factor. Especially
for men, I think.

It must strike at the very heart of their concept as the
strong, independent bread-winning leader of the family.

It did for my dad, anyway.

I thought I was prepared even if he wasn't.

I thought the family was prepared even if I turned out not
to be.

I had given everyone ample warning and instructions. All of
the granddaughters had come to the home prior to this day to

meet the director and check it out. They all knew that it was just getting too difficult for me to care for Dad's personal hygiene needs. Because of my years as a caregiver, I was not bothered in the least by this aspect of his care, but he adamantly refused to let me help him, as he refused to admit that he needed such help. I know it was embarrassing for him, and any suggestion of outside help triggered such negative behaviour that I had to consider the option of a nursing home.

Then July 11th happened.

Moving day had arrived.

The day I dreaded.

The day I needed so badly.

The day my dad dreaded but didn't realize he needed so badly.

He had no clue that this day had arrived . . . in my later journals I referred to this day as "the big mistake on July 11, 2007."

There actually are no journals between July 9th and July 14th.

It was such an emotional nightmare that I couldn't even write about it.

In spite of my best-laid plans, it was awful!

I tried to remain positive and cheerful, tried to be a pillar of strength for him and for the family with, I hoped, a bit left over for myself. His doctor had given me a small dose of lorazepam to help keep him calm on the hour-long drive to the home. It was not a medication he was used to, though. It affected him poorly so that he peed himself at the family lunch I had planned as a show of support for the event.

This, of course, deeply embarrassed my dad and fuelled his defensiveness so that all of the grandchildren fell prey to shame and guilt for participating. When we arrived at the home he called them traitors, bastards, enemies, any name that he could think of to lash out in anger and fear.

He could not have known how much homework I had done.

It was a home chosen specifically because it offered him some freedom of movement. It was a nice little bachelor-type apartment in a home with a library and little cafés within walking distance so we could continue to enjoy our dinner dates. There was also a leash-free park close by to walk the dogs when I brought them for a visit.

None of this mattered to him, though, and within just a day, he had a complete breakdown.

I had never ever seen my dad so crestfallen, so dejected.

Then, one by one the family members also melted down, lost whatever emotional resolve they had, so that once again I was the "last man standing" to shoulder the responsibility.

Well, I lasted two days in that lonely hell, and then I also caved and "rescued" my dad from the home.

The director of the home was not pleased with me. He tried to convince me to leave my dad there for two weeks without visiting to give him a chance to adjust on his own.

I just could not do that.

I took him up to my brother's cottage for a vacation away from the mess and madness of it all, and as the journals will attest, this was a welcome respite for both of us. With my brother's help, it offered a restorative environment in which to regroup and rethink the whole "damn home" thing.

Journal Entry: July 15, 2007

Well I'm grateful to be here.

I'm still a bit angry though.

What the hell happened last week?

I guess I acted poorly, but I couldn't stand that look on his face.

He looked abandoned for God's sake. What was I supposed to do? Walk away?

No one wants to talk about it, so I don't.

I feel like I let everyone down, but I'm kinda numb still so . . .

Dad doesn't seem to remember anything about it, which is good I suppose.

At least he is happy here at the cottage.

I am too because I have Ron's help during the night if Dad needs to go to the bathroom.

I know we can't stay here indefinitely.

No one wants to talk about that either.

This whole damn home thing.

That's fine with me.

It's a beautiful day to take Dad out in the boat.

Ron calls him "Pops."

I like that.

Journal Entry: July 25, 2007

I love the mornings here.

This is the best rest I have had in such a long time.

Dad is much more relaxed here, too.

I think that old house triggered a lot of his anger.

His sorrow, too.

He asks about his old home every day, and all I say is that the neighbours are taking care of it.

Guess I'll have to go there soon.

Make a decision of some sort.

We are all going to an auction tonight!

Yah!

A Tall Fish Tale

After the big mistake on July 11th, my dad and I spent an enjoyable and relatively stress-free summer at my brother's cottage. Since going backwards was not an option, I started to make plans for us to move forward, which meant eventually finding a place for my dad and me to live together again, closer to my family and friends.

In the meantime, we settled into cottage life like we had been doing for the past few summers.

This passage was so much easier for me because I had Ron's help during the day, and if the night had been rough, I could take an afternoon nap and renew my strength.

Dad was more content here as well and sat most days on a couch looking out onto the lake enjoying the plethora of vacation activities that constantly dotted the water.

My dad had been an avid fisherman all his life and a great proponent of catch and release, long before it was widely accepted. He had fished countless lakes in Canada from coast to coast, and he had as many stories—yes fish stories. But his most animated and passionate ones were always about his experiences with other fishermen who kept everything they caught and didn't have the vision to release what they wouldn't eat or share. It was a hot topic for him indeed.

By this time though, he had grown wary of going out in the boat to fish, so when he did cast off it was just at the end of the dock. And there were days he didn't even want to fish, because he said he felt sorry for the fish. I thought it curious at the time, but later wondered if he felt an affinity with the fish, an affinity to being snagged unexpectedly by some unseen force and dragged into another dimension against his will.

Well, not only was my dad a great storyteller, but he was also a great story maker, and he didn't let us down in this last summer. One afternoon, we heard shouts of, "Help! Help!" coming from the dock, coming from my dad.

My heart dropped, of course, and I went running down the yard to save him.

Ron beat me to it, and when I arrived I saw the two of them holding on to dad's fishing rod reefing it into a perfect C. That's when I noticed the bend in the rod was not down towards the water but up towards the sky.

Ron was hysterical with laughter as he helped the old fisherman reel in his catch, as it flew and swooped and tried to get away.

"Poor old seagull," my dad kept saying.

The Sad Residue
of His Losses

And so it was that in the fall of 2007, we resumed our funny little life together in a rented house outside Guelph. I had trepidation about trying again, of course, but with the added bonus of being in my hometown, I embarked on this new chapter with hope.

It was still difficult, but there were many moments of joy and goodwill with the love and support of friends and family so close by.

My daughter became my dad's constant companion for much of this year, which allowed me to return to work part time. This was a great relief, not only because it got me out of the house and interacting with others, but also because it gave my dad a break from me too. My daughter was wonderful with him, and he behaved most of the time when they were together.

Years later, she would say that this time was so precious because hearing his wonderful stories over and over again gave her the advantage of remembering them in detail, something that would not have happened if she had only seen him once in a while.

We settled into the new surroundings well enough. It wasn't easy to find a home to rent that allowed us to keep our two dogs, but, eventually, I did find one out in the country. It took my dad a short period of time to adjust, because it was so quiet and away from the hubbub that had surrounded his home in the city. However, I had always found peace in being in natural surroundings and hoped the serenity of a country setting would ease his agitated mind.

And indeed we both were refreshed and content throughout the first few months. We could walk the dogs down the lane without leashing them, and we were minutes away from friends as well as a multitude of new dining spots to explore. I registered him in an "out and about" group in a town nearby, and the house was large enough to accommodate overnight guests should anyone from out of town come to visit.

The house itself was well off the road, which suited me fine. I knew that any escapes that my dad might plan would be thwarted by his own fragile stamina on the long walk down the endless, winding driveway.

Although I knew he missed the busy city surroundings, I was able to capture his attention and imagination with peanuts scattered all over the back deck. This one act alone created a cacophony of social activity for him to watch, from greedy jays and other hungry birds to squirrels and chipmunks scampering nonstop up the railing, across the ledge, and on out into the field. If his eyesight had allowed, he would have been able to see the shadows of the deer moving through the twilight across the fields as well. He knew they were there, though, by the anxious panting it caused in the dogs at his feet.

Because we were close to friends, we were able to host card get-togethers on Friday nights, a thoroughly enjoyable time for both of us.

Even my journals became more positive in the first few months, and it did seem like we had established a winning situation for both of us.

Sadly though, as the late fall weather settled in, and the skies darkened in preparation for winter, we stayed indoors more often. His mood began to darken as well. He did not approve of this new "prison," and he treated all who came to help us to a healthy dose of his displeasure with everything.

I gave substantial thought to this in the ensuing years, and, eventually, it occurred to me that he aimed this habitual annoyance at me, not only because I was the one who took him from his home, but also because I looked increasingly like my mom and reminded him of all he had lost since her death. He didn't see it this way, of course. He just felt the sad residue of his losses as a persistent low-grade irritation.

Still, he was welcomed into the community of my daughter's friends, as well as mine, with overwhelming open arms, and, in the end, no one ever said they were less than blessed by coming to know this man, as frustrated and ornery as he grew daily.

Journal Entry: September 12, 2007

It is blissfully peaceful and quiet here in the mornings.

I love the sounds of the birds in the trees and the farm sounds in the distance.

Dad is struggling with that a bit. He said there is nothing to look at out the window, so we bought a bag of peanuts, and now there are tons of birds and squirrels on the back porch for him to watch.

He really seems to enjoy that.

It will be good as long as he doesn't let the killer cat out.

I know he knows that, but will he remember that he knows that?

We had a lovely card game last night with Ron and Louise.

Dad needs a bit of help with the game now but he tells stories the whole time anyway, so it's fun and entertaining nonetheless.

I am always amazed when he pulls a new one I've never heard before out of his hat.

Funny, he can't remember something he did two seconds earlier, but he has a razor-sharp mind for the details of stories from long ago.

Journal Entry: November 3, 2007

Thought I should write sometimes at night after the day is done and my well-meant attempts for the day are behind me.

The mornings are usually so innocent and un-ruffled it seems, and I am inspired to hope for the day ahead.

The night with its weary moon shadows certainly finds me in a different frame of mind.

Though I try to give my dad the best of my attention and care, he is never satisfied and exhausts me beyond words. However, he has gone to bed now, and, even though I am cross-eyed with fatigue, I appreciate these few moments of candlelight and quiet music to spend with my own contemplations and aloneness.

Dad was already up and about when I tried to write this morning, and it was impossible.

I find sometimes I write simply to get away from his endless suffocating bid for my full attention.

He loves to read; he loves to watch television; he

loves to watch the birds on the deck . . . why can't he leave me alone for two minutes?

Anyway, he's not even here now, and still I go on about this . . .

Journal Entry: November 19, 2007

Such a sweet gentle house and home had been created here, but once again I feel unsure and unsafe with my decision to bring Dad here.

He has a very bad cold and no wonder.

I have found him outside on the deck with his dog twice this week without a shirt on.

Oh God, does he really need to be in a home where someone can watch him every minute?

What does it require to care for him?

I guess I thought loving him was enough.

But now I am starting to feel fear.

And anger again.

I went to bed angry last night, because he let the cat out in the freezing cold and forgot he did it two seconds later!

Then he denied it, and we argued over that.

His confusion and denial drive me up the wall.

I know this is a big lesson for me in patience and kindness.

My fear is that I'm failing the class

Failing my dad.

Journal Entry: December 11, 2007

In so many ways, this move to Guelph was the perfect thing to do.

Too bad I lost some family members overboard on the journey to get here.

Well, at least I can sleep at night knowing full well I didn't push them out.

They jumped freely by their own choice.

What's sad is that my dad doesn't even ask about anyone anymore.

If they don't come around, he doesn't know they exist.

He asks about his house, though.

All I care to do is get through the winter with extracurricular activities and see what the spring brings.

Anything can happen at this point, it seems.

Journal Entry: May 14, 2008

Dad was up wandering with his flashlight into the wee hours of the morning.

Again.

He came into my room three or four times and flicked on the light.

Apparently, he was looking for the geek who was trying to make him have a bath.

I tried hard to convince him that we are the only two people in the house.

I have to work this morning . . . this is exhausting.

Not sure if I'm in for a breakdown or a breakthrough.

A crackup or a crackdown.

Dad's need for attention has jumped the scale.

Again.

Journal Entry: May 20, 2008

Just two more weeks 'til Dad goes to the cottage, and I begin to pack yet again.

I feel so deeply lonely, it is almost unbearable.

But it doesn't feel like it is for another person.

Who then?

I think I am lonely for myself and that sounds crazy.

Thank God no one else reads this stuff.

I feel a strange fear looming around the idea of not having Dad for company anymore.

I fear that when he goes away and I don't have the routine of caring for him I just won't be anyone anymore.

Or I won't know who to be, if it's just me.

This kind of thinking gives me the willies, I swear.

I've got laundry to do.

A Move to the Veterans Centre

By May of 2008, as much as I tried to remain understanding and strong, I eventually had to admit I was just no longer able to give my dad the care he needed.

Because he was a war vet, the VAC (Veterans Affairs Canada) had approached him years earlier with information about his eligibility for a place in the Sunnybrook Veterans Centre in Toronto.

I wasn't happy with the idea of him being so far away from me, but my brother and I decided to investigate this option anyway.

I was torn by what the facility offered.

The building where the home is located is an extension of the Sunnybrook Health Sciences Centre, a hospital, so it has an institutional look to it. The secure wing my dad would be in was itself quite hospital like, with no carpets, no curtains—very functional but not very homey.

What won me over, though, was the lovely and spacious garden courtyard that is accessible to those in the secure wing. That meant during the warm months my dad could come and go into the garden as he pleased. The garden perimeter was secure, so the door from his wing was not locked. I also considered that he would be with other old vets who shared something powerful in common with his early years—the war. And it was exactly halfway between where my brother lived in Peterborough and where I lived in Guelph.

This time, the move was less dramatic. My brother had his room set up before we arrived and only the two of us accompanied him. If I'd learned anything from the "big mistake on July 11th," it was that my dad needed this transition to be private and uneventful.

This time, I also heeded the advice of the charge nurse and did not go to visit or interfere for two weeks, to give him the chance to adjust on his own terms. I kept in touch daily with the caregivers, and then when the two weeks had passed I started to visit him regularly and take him "out on the town" as the other gentlemen liked to quip.

We would go to the leash-free dog park on the hospital property, and it didn't take us long to find a few favourite watering holes with servers that always welcomed us with smiles and cheers.

Thus, it was not long before there was a return of peace between us, and I was so grateful for that. I could once again enjoy our time together, as could he, and our mutual laughter eventually returned over many lazy luncheons and dog walks.

Because I was looking after my grandson, I would bring him with me on my weekly trips to the city to see Dad. These were delightful occasions. Everyone in the wing, staff and resident alike, fawned over his great-grandson, and he was so proud to waltz down the hall with the little man perched atop his walker.

We set up a bird feeder just outside his window and made it a kind of mission to replenish it every week when I came to visit. Eventually, we were filling all the birdfeeders around the courtyard, and Dad thoroughly enjoyed this philanthropic project.

But, since it was an entire day's journey to get into the city and take him out for lunch (with rush hour an all), I could only come to visit once a week, sometimes twice. I wasn't pleased with this, but I had to be satisfied, knowing there were excursions for the Vets and lots of activities he could participate in for company. And he did.

However, when the time came that he couldn't participate any more, he became depressed, so my brother and I decided to move him to a home closer to me where I could visit him more often. We were not encouraged to make this decision, though, and were warned that another move could weaken his fragile health.

But I knew he needed to be closer to me, and he was happy at this news too.

Journal Entry: December 12, 2008

If only Dad lived closer.

I'm not fond of the drive across the GTA when the weather is like this.

But I promised I would come, and I can't bear the thought that he would be so disappointed if I didn't show.

It's a funny thought, really.

He usually says he didn't know I was coming even though he has been told.

Oh well . . .

It'll be good to see him.

Good to hit the pub and share a few giggles.

He is so sweet now.

I don't like to see him cry when I leave, though.

I wish they didn't have to have such big metal doors that close off his section.

I feel like I'm closing prison doors when I leave.

I thought I'd feel relieved when he went to Sunnybrook.

Ron says I worry too much.

Journal Entry: July 29, 2009

Dad is looking pretty frail these days.

I had hoped the warm weather and the gardens would cheer him up like last year.

He is not as social as he used to be.

Not when I see him, anyway.

Apparently he regales the nurses with his battle-field adventures, though.

What a character.

I don't want to tell them he never went overseas.

I don't want to pop his balloon, spoil his party!

Am starting to think about moving him closer to me.

No doubt the family will not be impressed, again.

I could be doing this all wrong, I know, but I have to follow my gut instinct.

I have to follow my conscience.

Don't I?

Best Jump I Ever Made

Usually, there is a very long waiting list for beds in nursing homes, but, as good fortune would have it, one opened up within a few months in a nursing home in the small picturesque town of Fergus, Ontario. What serendipity, since this town was only minutes away from the house we had rented in Guelph two years prior, so we already knew the parks and pubs well.

I was able to find a beautiful little apartment for myself just around the corner from the home, and, with the extra visits from me and friends and family, he once again rallied, and his good spirits returned.

His second floor window overlooked the parking lot, and

when I had to leave he could wave at me as I got into my car. He knew that I lived just around the corner, and this seemed to give him great comfort, and as his need for security increased I simply told him I had an apartment on the first floor of his building.

My dad had never been a snoopy type of guy, but here he loved to watch the comings and goings down in the parking lot and took his sentinel post at the window quite seriously.

Although this move was initially arranged so that I could see my dad more often, it turned out to be a blessing in ways I hadn't expected.

Ironically, and without planning, it was the best jump we ever made!

This home was remarkable.

On the surface, it did not appear to have the advantages, or so-called "bells and whistles" of some larger establishments, but it had the best of the best resource: staff who were seasoned with experience and genuine caring.

This was very important for my dad's care. Even as he was losing his mental judgment, his emotional nature was still keen, and he needed the depth of understanding and empathy that so many of these remarkable women offered.

My "Smitty Story" later in this section is an example of that.

And there were countless other aspects to this home that

made it superior to the institution he had been in. The dining room was smaller and consequently more personable. The home was small enough that the charge nurse on his floor as well as the director of the entire home was accessible when I had concerns or ideas to share. I rarely had to make an appointment for weeks in advance. The laundry was done on a small scale, and he didn't lose clothes regularly. I could also come and take him out for dinner, and he would be ready because the message I sent actually reached his caregiver and didn't get lost in a shift change or large chain of communication.

The neighbourly hospitality that is characteristic of this small town infused the home, while its picturesque surroundings so close to the park along the river afforded a refreshing change from the frenetic overstimulation of the big city.

While he was still able, it was easy to take him out to stroll along the riverbank, and as it was reminiscent of our dog walks in the woods years earlier, he welcomed the serenity it offered.

As did I.

Journal Entry: August 21, 2010

It is so wonderful to be able to rise in the quiet of this new apartment.

From up here on the hill, I can hear the geese gathering on the river below.

It puts me in an otherworldly frame of mind.

I'm glad the fall-down, break-apart, shattered-on-the-ground part is over.

But the reconstruction has not started yet.

Dad moves into the new home on Monday, and I feel myself bracing for . . .

Impact.

For some reason, I am suddenly uncertain of my decision, fearing a failure will bring new criticism from the family.

Oh well, it is in motion now, and Dad and I will make the best of it as we have always done.

I feel bad moving him again, but I know he recognizes me as a constant in all this shuffling.

He still recognizes me, so I'll go with that for now.

Journal Entry: May 24, 2012

This morning is like a space out of time.
All the customary activities await me:
Going to work and visiting my dad.

Yet this sanctuary I call home, with its beautiful
and gentle breeze tickling the patio foliage
And my ankles
Tell me to relish this moment because it is so fleet-
ing
Like life itself.

I hope Dad will eat the raspberries I picked for him.
Guess I'll go early and catch him awake.

Let Me Tell You About Smitty: A PSW Story

There are so many people involved in the life of a person with Alzheimer's, and often one will stand out clearly: a champion of a sort. Someone who "gets it" in a way that no one else can. I'm sure for many this is a family member (as some considered me in the beginning), but for so many more of us it turns out to be a professional caregiver, or perhaps a community care worker, who shines through the veil of sadness and saves a day or two.

My dad's mental and physical condition took a substantial downturn in the last two years of his life. He was in his early 90s, after all, and had fared amazingly well for the 10 years he had lived with the diagnosis of Alzheimer's.

Even as much as his mental collapse was a daily challenge, it was the difficulty with his personal hygiene that finally led to the decision to give him into the care of a nursing home. He just didn't realize that he needed help and found any attempt to assist him embarrassing and aggravating. In the last year, this was difficult even for the professional caregivers at the home. But, as I have already mentioned, the home he settled in had mostly good ol' fashioned caregivers: those who were grandfathered in when the compulsory accreditation for Personal Support Workers became part of the system.

They weren't just good; they were remarkable. What they said and did with the residents came from years of experience and authentic caring, not from a college course, however sincerely earned.

There was one woman in particular there who instantly took to my dad, and, since her last name was Smith as well, they became fast friends over the shared nickname and secret brotherhood of being a "Smitty."

She could get him to do things, like bathe, or eat, or take his pills, or stop screaming obscenities into the hall when no one else could.

He honestly wanted to please her, because they were Smitty bonded.

I remember well the day I got the call that he had bitten her and sent her to the hospital. They had to let me know this had happened as part of the protocol, of course.

I felt awful and was quick to apologize to her, but she remained totally calm and reminded me that it was not personal, and that it wasn't even my dad who had caused this injury, it was the illness. I knew she didn't take it personally, because she knew my dad didn't mean to hurt anyone, especially her.

I knew she was not only right, but kind as well.

Then the next call came a few months later to inform me that he had head-butted her and knocked her out cold!

The administrator had no choice but to move Smitty to another wing of the facility so that she was no longer one of his primary caregivers. Still, she continued to visit him and clown around with him and help calm him down when she was needed.

The night he passed, this wonderful woman came to his room to pay her respects before going home for Christmas Eve. We cried together, and I really felt like I was with a sister.

In the course of writing this book, I found myself more and more frequently in conversations with others who have either gone through, or are currently going through, the passage of caring for a parent with Alzheimer's. Even the stats I am familiar with hadn't prepared me for discovering how many of us share this experience. But I have also found through these individual stories that there is quite a broad spectrum of experiences. This is because Alzheimer's, by its own great mysterious nature, can affect its victims in so many different ways. And yet, as true as this may be, there do seem to be two distinct streams in this continuum.

There are those whose behaviour becomes very docile and whose attention, such as it is, can be directed and easily managed, in spite of the mental decline. There is a gentleness to their unravelling.

And then there are those whose behaviours are volatile, aggressive, moody, and unpredictable to boot.

That was my dad.

He had a heart of gold, and yet his unravelling exposed the raw nerves of every disappointment and irritation that had dogged his life.

Thank goodness there were caregivers such as this remarkable woman to see the Smitty still inside of him and honour the man he now rarely knew he was.

Part Five

Finding Healing in the Journey

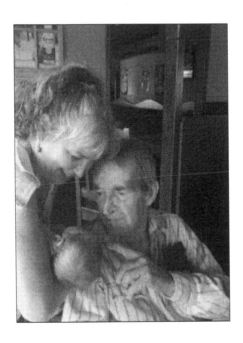

What Is Memory?

As I mentioned in the introduction, long before I accepted the role of caring for my dad 24/7, I worked as a caregiver in nursing homes for many years, primarily in the secure wings where the patients were suffering from one form of dementia or another.

At this time, I was also active as a stage artist/singer songwriter.

At one point, because of my observation and emotional involvement in this caregiving field, I was inspired to write a song based on a heartfelt inquiry about this illness. The song is called "I Remember," and it was written to challenge the focus on the forgetting aspect of dementia and ask, what is it, if anything, that can never be forgotten?

Near the end of my dad's battle with Alzheimer's, I was visiting him one evening and sitting quietly at his bedside giving him a treatment of Therapeutic Touch/Reiki, since I had recently acquired my practitioner level two for this energy work.

I wasn't actually touching him but rather stroking the energy around his head.

The room was calm, and I was quite enjoying the sense of being close to him, even though he had been unresponsive for days and days.

Then out of the blue, as a total surprise to me, he yelled out, "Sharon, stop dancing on my head!"

It surprised the hell out of me. I had long stopped hoping for any personal recognition of who I was, and I had no idea he even knew I was there!

What was happening?

Who was yelling out my name?

Where was he really?

I know that when we read to some victims of coma, they are able to hear us, sense us, even if they cannot acknowledge it. Is it so different for other brain injury victims?

My dad responded from somewhere!

With all of the details of his personal story disappearing, did he still recognize my energy?

My touch?

My smell?

This made such an impression on me, because it is the very idea I had tried to express many years earlier in that song.

There was another moment in my life where this idea hit home. Months after my dad had passed, I received a text from Melody, the same niece who had held vigil with me on the night of his passing.

Quite out of the blue she asked, "Did you know that your name came from Grampa's favourite song?"

"Ah, no," I replied. "I was always under the impression that my name came from my godmother."

"No," she said. "Grampa sang this all the time!"

Then she sent me a link to a song recorded in 1924, a song by a man named Whispering Jack Smith, a song called Cecelia!

"WHAT?" I yelled over text as I pressed play to the link she had sent.

Then the song began, and I started to cry. I was truly shocked that from somewhere deep and old inside me I recognized that song!

I did not *remember* that song. It was a feeling more penetrating, more visceral, even more ancient than that. It was a type of presence, an essence, a sense of being very, very little and hearing this song over and over.

And it evoked an emotion I have no name for.

It was tender, and sweet, and explosive at the same time.

Yet it was not what I would call a memory.

What type of recall was this? I asked.

Much more important, though, are the questions, like:

Was my dad experiencing this same type of feeling about old experiences in his own life?

Was his a similar recall that did not involve the mind so much as some other sense?

Was he remembering things he could not express because he had no way to describe them?

In short, are there types of recall that do not belong to the mind primarily?

I hope this will be the next horizon over which we peer in our search for understanding Alzheimer's, focusing not so much on what is not remembered, but more on what can truly never be forgotten. I think the current trend of music therapy acknowledges that music falls in that category. I think it is a good step in the right direction.

Perhaps we will also begin to consider the Soul and how its memory abides through the experience of Alzheimer's.

I REMEMBER

So you think that I have forgotten
All the times we were given to share
Well it's you who are failing to notice
When no other was there,
The smell of your hair;
I remember the smell of your hair

How I wish that you could come over
To the place where I am fading away
It's been so long, I'd like you to stay awhile
For no one can replace
The smile on your face;
I remember the smile on your face

Everyone has things to remember
It's all part of the master plan
I'll remind you, the next time you are over
That I still understand
The touch of your hand;
I remember the touch of your hand.[1]

---

1   "I Remember" © 2000 Sharon Cecelia Smith
To listen to the song visit asilentbugle.com

Revelation

"The events in our lives happen in a sequence in time, but in their significance to ourselves they find their own order . . . the continuous thread of revelation."

—Eudora Welty, One Writer's Beginnings[3]

There were two purposes I felt I had as my dad's caregiver. One was the quite obvious role of being his protector and helpmate, and the other, I can see now, derived from this beautiful idea that American author Eudora Welty penned in her book *One Writer's Beginnings*.

It was very important to me to try to understand what was happening in my life from the perspective of a greater purpose and the potential of each experience to offer a revelation of some kind. Being the far-sighted thinker that he was, my dad had always encouraged me to see things, especially problems, within the context of a larger picture, a greater plan, a meaningful vision. And so I was always on the alert for "aha moments" with him, and this purpose gave me great stamina for the distance we travelled. I suppose this is why I journaled faithfully every day as well . . . lest I too one day would forget the small but significant revelations of our precious time together.

Strangely though, so many of the revelations have come long after I wrote the journals. It has been in the rereading of them all these years later that I can see insights dawning in the words. Insights I didn't always acknowledge or realize at the time.

Some of the revelations happened in spite of me, I have to admit. They happened without warning.

Some of them were personal and came out spontaneously in the journals, while others had to do with me allowing the moment to be whatever reality my dad needed.

It wasn't only the hat and the stuffed dog (from Part One) that appeared out of nowhere, it was also my ability to see a fresh way, a kind way of responding to my dad's fractured perspective.

I guess what I have called *revelations* are perhaps simply moments that have inspired my willingness to surrender.

Journal Entry: August 1, 2004

The morning glories are beautiful today, Mom.

Purple, magenta, pink, royal blue, white.

I wish you could have seen them as they are now.

More beautiful than ever since you passed away.

And the dolphin wind chimes we bought are lovely too.

Last week I heard Dad say to the doctor,

"When she's alive, your wife is just your wife.

But when she dies, she becomes everything."

Kind of made me look at my dad in another way.

Did he realize how profound that was?

Or is the simple truth just that profound?

Is that you, Mom?

The wind sings to me in chimes that dangle lazily from the awning.

One note plays a delicate repetition as another joins in.

And the dolphins dance to and fro on their plumb line.

From around the corner come the garden

chimes, deep and resonant.

A pas de deux for a moment's listening pleasure.

And then the wind moves on.

Are you riding its passage past my door Mom?

Journal Entry: March 9, 2007

I have become silent over the issue of my struggle between my own needs and those of Papa.

I am not thriving, just barely surviving in his home here.

I have stayed on a year after the first real cry for release that happened last spring.

I have stayed on and normalized a painful situation for many reasons.

I have blamed my dad's behaviour for my fatigue and indifference.

But I am sensing more is happening here.

It is my inability to change that has the situation stagnant.

What am I afraid of, really?

Being single again?

Being alone again?

I have told myself that I stay with him so he will not feel abandoned.

But that's not altogether true.

I don't want to be abandoned either.

I think I fear that if I do this to him, one day I will be abandoned by my children.

What goes around comes around as they say.

Abandonment issues are so hard for me to look at.

Even now I want to look away from these words.

I feel kind of sick, crazy, maybe.

Journal Entry: January 23, 2008

So hard to get up on these cold dark mornings.

I am a mess of emotions these days.

I am feeling burned out again with Dad, and he seems to have no end of energy to follow me around the house all day long. Sometimes, I think he is trying to torture me into taking him back to his home.

I can't go anywhere in the house that he doesn't follow immediately.

It is torture whether he means it or not.

And the family is nowhere to be found.

I hate being so bitter, really I do.

It must be so lonely for Papa when he can't read any more or do anything for himself.

He was always such an independent guy.

A natural born bachelor as mom liked to say.

I am so grateful for these kind thoughts.

They rescue me from my own misery.

Oh!

Two deer just passed by in the field close to the house.

They look so gentle but they must be so strong to survive the winter out there.

So gentle and so strong . . . okay, okay, I get it.

Journal Entry: February 29, 2008

I have known moments of mental clarity in my life,
but what I feel this morning is different.

 This one has nothing to do with feeling smart
or right.

  I just woke up this morning with a kind of "aha."

  I've been dreading the thought of moving my dad
into a home.

  It's not a thought anymore.

  I see that it must be.

  It's a breakthrough.

Come waves

Break at my shore.

Waves of emotion that I have long kept away

Embrace me now that I may go forth

From this moment as a whole

And not a half in search of its other.

Journal Entry: December 13, 2004

I am trying to stay so cheerful for my dad.

Maybe I shouldn't listen to the news.

A world of murder, and poison, and hate, and lies.

So sad.

The angels themselves must cry.

Children are caught in the black sweep of human suffering.

I really must stop listening to the news.

WAILING OF ANGELS

Out of the white noise

Above the city's roar

Behind the static of the global grid

Surrounding the whirl of the great wind turbines

Hidden in the hush of the mountaintop forests

Sprawled across the burning sands of arid earth

Slicing the vastness of the ocean's mystery

With pristine sonics we cannot hear

With human ears,

A sound lives and moves

It is the wailing of angels

Deep, sad, wise sobs

Crystal beings crying in the heart of God

God's eye

Watchful

Ancient

Like whales

The Lowly Morning Glory

For as long as I can remember, I have adored morning glories.

I developed a fierce loyalty to them long before I began to understand my attraction.

To assuage this deep fascination, I began to photograph them while Dad and I were still living in his home.

I remember feeling guilty one morning for letting them transport me to a place in my heart and mind so far away from the suffering and irritation of the daily news, so far away from the stress and anxiety of my daily life with my dad.

Was I irresponsible for escaping from the cares and concerns of the world by giving myself so completely to the simple beauty of a flower?

And the next question was . . . Did I even have a choice?

My attraction was so strong I didn't feel like I had a choice.

On the first anniversary of my mom's passing, I was sitting on the patio writing in my journals when one of my earrings fell down under the lip of the garden fence that was covered with morning glory vines. As I descended on hands and knees down into the clot of grasses and weedy vines gone amuck to retrieve it, I discovered something so profound it had the effect of a great knock on the head.

To my delight and surprise, I spotted the brilliant flash of a magenta morning glory! As perfect a morning glory as any that bloomed up the fence in full view of the sun, or of the sky, or of the admiring glances from members of the neighbourhood strolling by.

It was astonishing to me.

Who would have ever noticed or admired this lovely, lovely sculpture down there, growing quietly at the bottom of the garden, if I hadn't seen it?

Why was it so lovely, so perfect?

So hidden and alone?

Blooming?

Beautifully content?

That little flower suddenly turned into a hero for me.

A kind of symbol of what I could be.

Journal Entry: July 3, 2005

Today is sad.

Sad for so many reasons.

Today I feel invisible but not in a good way.

It's a lonely, bitter, "who gives a shit" kind of invisibility.

Puzzling really, because in all honesty I generally like the anonymity of being dad's sidekick.

He gets all the attention, and I am usually so tired I don't want it anyway.

I don't feel particularly entertaining these days.

It's not the public attention I miss.

I miss some kind of appreciation from my family ... no one ever says, "Good job, Sharon."

Or, "How are you holding up, Sharon?"

Mom would if she was here.

I miss Mom.

Oh my ...

THE LOWLY MORNING GLORY

Oh Gracious flower

You stun me with your natural radiance

Blooming as you dare to do in mottled light

You should be in the spotlight

Yet you shine in the wings of this garden perfor-

mance.

And I who attend the show applaud your humble

beauty

And wisdom

A very strange sense of peace and strength is

upon me, and deeper into love have I now fallen with

the lowly morning glory.

One Day at a Time

At least once in our lives, we have all come across a saying or written phrase from a favourite novel, perhaps a poem, or a movie that affects us deeply, stays with us through the years, and even gets quoted when we are waxing philosophical—a saying that alters the way we think about something or someone, perhaps even expands our understanding of life itself.

It might be a prayer that comes to our aid in a time of crisis or a simple song lyric that evokes a happy memory to lighten an emotional burden.

For me, the Serenity Prayer is one such touchstone.

"God grant me the serenity to accept the things I

cannot change,

Courage to change the things I can,

And wisdom to know the difference."⁴

Although I didn't consciously see it at the time, it is clear now that many of my journals were written with this Prayer dancing invisibly behind the words.

For a number of years back in the 1980s, I had been quite active in a twelve-step program called Al-Anon. This program, as it is commonly known now, is designed for people living with a significant other, be it a spouse, a close family member, or a dear friend who suffers from addiction.

As I mentioned in "It's a Family Affair" (Part Three) Alzheimer's has an affinity with the mental illness of addiction in its traumatic effect on other family members.

During particularly difficult bouts with my dad I found myself reaching for the solace that I found in two little books still in my library from those earlier Al-Anon days. One is called *Courage to Change*, by the Al-Anon Family Group Headquarters, Inc., and is named after this beloved Serenity Prayer.

My mom, many, many years earlier had often quoted this prayer as well, and no doubt that had seeded its impact on me.

It is a prayer that has been invoked daily all over the world for many years, and I drew strength from knowing this as much as from the power of its message. Every day there simply was nothing I needed more than acceptance, and courage, and wisdom to stay the distance with my dad.

The other book is called *One Day at a Time in Al-Anon*, also by the Al-Anon Family Group Headquarters, Inc., and, named, of course, after the arch slogan of all twelve-step philosophies. I found encouragement in the well-worn advice that this slogan offers, and strength in the daily affirmations and testimonials for self-care. These stories came from those who have had the personal experience of needing this deep advice to live, tackle, appreciate, and embrace life one day at a time, with tempered courage and wisdom. I was so influenced by this line of thinking that, with only a few exceptions, my daily journaling was not so much a diary of specific issues with my dad as it was a way of writing myself into this healthy mindset.

Journal Entry: January 11, 2008

Feeling a deep protective compassion for my dad today.

Sense of how brave he is trying to be with this huge change.

Sense of how scared he is of being alone, being abandoned.

Sense of how unfair it has been of me to blame him for my struggles with his illness.

I want him to feel safe here with me.

I don't want to be angry anymore at this cruel disease that is stealing him away from me.

Angry at my inability to help him stay.

Angry at the constant reminder that I am as powerless as he is.

My dad doesn't deserve to be around my anger.

I want to change.

Journal Entry: April 8, 2008

Cried myself to sleep last night.

A sad movie pulled out more tears than the plot called for.

Realized as I was snuffling under the covers that I was crying for my dad.

Sad little Papa.

I thought I could infuse some joy into his life by moving to a peaceful setting in the country.

I thought the serenity here would save us.

But his condition has continued to decline, and he is not at all happy here.

My attitude about caring for him has also declined, and I cannot help myself.

I ignore him to survive his suffocating need for attention.

And now I have added a plan to move again to this complicated cocktail of woe.

Perhaps spring will bring some renewal for us both.

The deer have returned to the fields.

Six of them.

Where is the seventh?

Lost in the woods over the winter, I guess.

Like parts of my dad.

Or

Parts of me.

In the End It Did Not Matter

The things that I did with and for my dad in the final few months of his decline were as much for my benefit as for his. I had finally learned to include my own well-being in the equation of our shrinking world together.

When we could no longer go out to enjoy a lunch, I would order drive-thru, and we'd park at the river and watch the boats go by, or the fishermen whip their fly rods gracefully to and fro down by the shallows.

When he could no longer get into the car for our outings, I would manoeuvre his wheelchair out onto the patio and have a picnic lunch, sometimes chasing the sunny spots two or three times as the light wove itself in and around the huge shade trees. On very hot days, we chased the shade instead.

When we could no longer go outside because of inclement weather, or because he was too agitated, I would sit with him in his room and watch old *Cisco Kid* videos or listen to Frank Sinatra songs on his CD player.

When he started to shut down completely and could no longer get out of bed or even open his eyes, I would sit beside his bed and stroke his brow and sing to him.

As my dad's capabilities dwindled away, I grabbed for any frayed thread I could reach to hold the fabric of our rapport together.

In the end it did not matter what we did, though.

A matter of pure presence wove its magic around our visits.

The Bridge Manoeuvre

In 2012, my daughter married a young man whose family was from Ottawa, but, sadly, Dad was not strong enough to make the trip to attend the wedding.

On the evening before the ceremony, we had gathered at the groom's parent's home after rehearsal, where his Mom, Lu-Anne and I were chatting about this and that. My dad's situation came up, and, in talking briefly about him, I mentioned that he had been stationed in Ottawa during the war, and that he repaired airplane instrument panels. She told me that her dad had been a pilot out of Ottawa during the same war.

"Oh," I said, "my dad says those young pilots were crazy!"

And I then proceeded to share with her one of my dad's favourite stories about the "bridge manoeuvre."

Between 1940–1945 during World War II, while my dad was stationed in Ottawa, part of his responsibility was to accompany each plane on a test flight after he had worked on it to make sure everything was functioning as it should be.

He was fond of telling the story of one young pilot whose name he couldn't remember, but who had decided to test my dad's nerve one day by flying the plane under a bridge right in Hawkesbury, a small town just outside of Ottawa.

My dad was none too pleased with this escapade, and, as he loved to whisper emphatically, he literally sh#t himself!

He always emphasized, however, that it wasn't so much a risk as it was a shock. He may have thought those guys were daredevils, but he acknowledged that they knew their aircrafts' capabilities like the backs of their hands. He trusted their judgment implicitly, but this was one memory never to be forgotten!

Well, wouldn't you know, this new family my daughter was marrying into also had a similar story! Except, their grandfather, whom they called Poppy, *was* the pilot who flew a plane one time and one time only under a bridge in Hawkesbury and scared the pants off of a fellow airman.

Was this a mysterious coincidence?

Was this just imaginative thinking?

So immediately Poppy was called and asked if the airman he had treated to the bridge manoeuvre those many years ago was named Frank Smith.

To which he candidly replied, "Oh my dear, they were all named Smith back in those days!"

It was bittersweet for me.

Sweet that the possibility of such a grand alignment should bless the vesper hour of my dad's storyline.

Bitter, that he was too far gone to appreciate the fantastic nature of it.

Irrespective of this, I told him later, "It's okay, Papa. I got this one."

Anticipatory Grief

"Anticipatory grief is the emotional pain of losing a loved one, felt in advance of the person's death. It's a common phenomenon among those who care for the terminally ill."[5]

—Paula Spencer Scott, in the Caring.com article, "Anticipatory Grief" ©

I remember well the first time I read the phrase "anticipatory grief."

I had a very bad reaction. I became irrationally angry, enraged actually.

I hated the sound of it, but, even more, I hated the very idea if it. I became a bit obsessed for a time, and my mind was drawn to it like a tongue to a jagged tooth. I couldn't stop thinking about it, each time summoning the same repulsion and anger. What nerve was it rubbing against?

This concept has surfaced again these many years later in my writing research and twigged my memory of this unusual response. I realize now that it was the very idea that anything about Alzheimer's could be anticipated that was so deeply offensive to me.

What triggered my dad's sudden mood swings was a mystery to me, and there was no way I could anticipate these moments.

One minute he was someone I recognized, and, in the blink of an eye, Alzheimer's voice would rip through his brain and come shooting out his mouth like a stray bullet.

I also resented the word grief. As far as I was concerned it had no place in a conversation about Alzheimer's. My dad was still alive, after all.

I believe now that if I had not had such a violent response to this concept it may actually have served to help me understand many of the emotions with which I was struggling.

But, no wonder my reaction was so volatile. It was defensive. And what I was defending was my refusal to grieve, my refusal to let go of my dad each time this happened, each time he disappeared a bit more into the void of unreachability.

I refused to grieve a little at a time, as this concept of anticipatory grief suggests.

Instead I froze.

Each time he slipped away a little more, I froze a little more and tightened my grip on him a little more.

Now ten years later, as I engage these memories, writing this book has been a difficult blessing as I discover hindsight revelations that will finally allow me to thaw, to let go, and to grieve at last.

Journal Entry: June 4, 2006

Boy, I'm in a mood today.

I am having a weird reaction to something I read yesterday.

It's an irrational reaction, really.

It's an idea someone has invented called *anticipatory grief* and the very sound of it makes me want to spit.

Who the hell thinks up these things, anyway?

Oh yeah, people who study them, not people who have them.

It offends me to be told how to feel about anything.

Especially this stuff with dad.

How dare someone name it anticipatory grief!

Anticipatory anything!

Piss off with your fancy names for this terrible feeling. As if it can be described and understood!

As if naming it gives it permission to be!

Journal Entry: November 4, 2007

I think I sit and write as much to contemplate as I do to document this journey with Dad.

Also to find a few moments respite from his suffocating bid for my attention.

And still my contemplations are all about him.

No wonder I feel trapped.

He just won't leave me alone for two seconds.

If he moved into a home, I'd have alone time.

God, even the thought of that gives me shivers.

Who's doing the trapping here, anyway?

What? Can't live with him, can't live without him?

Am I afraid to be alone if he goes into a home?

Or is it because I have worked in them and know how an old person can regress to the level of the group in there?

Ugh, that thought paralyzes me, too.

Sometimes I feel good about this idea
But not always.

Sometimes I feel brave about everything

But not always.

Sometimes I feel kind about this situation

But not always.

Sometimes I feel grateful to be with dad

But not always.

Guess I have Sometimer's.

Good grief!

The Forever Missing

It has been one of the most unusual aspects of writing this book, to experience the unexpected surfacing of grief, still raw, still unfinished.

The tears have come suddenly, randomly, and they have been searing.

I have found myself feeling very guilty and second-guessing decisions I had made ten years ago, second-guessing assumptions I had made about my dad's behaviour, second-guessing my reasons for looking after him all by myself in the first place.

And rage, pure and simple, for the sheer unfairness of it all.

I was sad when my dad passed but not with the intense

eruption of these feelings.

Grief is a difficult emotion to understand or process at any time, let alone years after the fact, after the experience, after the passing.

It is a journey unto itself.

To say that I was left depleted and weak after my dad passed is fair. I had no energy left to grieve, or even to write for that matter. It was only when I began reading the journals and understanding what was tucked in between the lines that the deep need to mourn came to the surface.

With the help of some wonderful bereavement counselling, I am coming to realize that it is simply part of the learning I continue to process in this journey with my dad.

I am grateful for this experience.

Grateful for this rite of passage through the pain of deep grieving to get to the tender embrace of the forever missing.

The Toast

Some say that the moment of death is not a coincidence, that somehow the person passing has a hand in the timing. After my dad passed, I began to wonder about this.

If this was indeed so, there did seem a number of reasons why he would choose Christmas Eve.

First of all, we all knew that he loved a good social gathering, and the little cocktail party we were having in his room that evening seemed a "Frankie" kind of exit. Not to mention that he would be assured of an honourary toast every Christmas Eve thereafter, since it was already a time of gathering and offering 'cheers'. And finally, my dad, always a frugal man, had often been called a "Scrooge," so this night was a fitting one on which to meet the phantoms of his life and be transformed!

But even later, as I further pondered the unique timing of his death, I came upon what I now consider to be the most probable reason for this night of all nights to be his last on earth. My Dad was afraid of very little in his life, certainly of no man. But the one thing I know he did have a respectful fear of was God, the almighty giver and taker of life.

We practiced grace on religious holidays and family gatherings, yet we were not avid churchgoers. He certainly acknowledged God, and the only exception to this absenteeism from conventional worship was Christmas Eve. For years and years, when I was in my teens, the one time we would go to church was Christmas Eve for the late night service—just the two of us.

I think he loved the music and pageantry of the ceremony and the simple tenderness of the Christmas story itself.

I also think he felt safe there.

He must have felt safe on that particular Christmas Eve in 2012. Safe enough to let go and commend his spirit into the hands of whatever benevolent Angel or shining star was attending to the Holy Birth.

And I'm pretty sure he knew there would be music. For on that night as no other, all over the world, voices would be raised in joyful chorus singing "Silent Night"!

A Silent Bugle

He died as he lived . . . making his presence count, marching along with the pageantry, a silent bugle to his lips.

Part Six

Journaling Questions and Inspiration

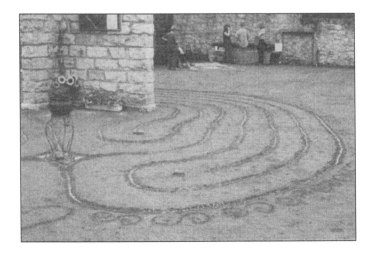

Journal Entry: April 20, 2005

Why do I write?

It isn't really for therapeutic reasons is it?

Unless it's therapeutic to do it just because it is something I do myself alone.

No one can read them except by invitation.

It's a privacy thing, a boundaries exercise, I guess.

I also harbour an idea that one day these journals will be useful in some way.

Maybe someone will find them and write a book.

Maybe my kids will find them interesting after I die.

I think I write to keep something stable in my life.

Like a platform to start the day, even if the rest of it goes all haywire.

Journal Entry: May 18, 2006

I find some mornings that this ritual of writing is not so much about having or not having anything to say . . .

It is about private time with myself, uninterrupted.

It is a time to simply feel the pulse of my own lonely gripe.

It is also a bit like sitting on the runway of my flight path.

Idling before takeoff into the skies of my daily life with my dad.

Sometimes it is a grace period in which I have to talk myself into taking off at all.

To gather the wind beneath my wings.

I am asking only for mercy and compassion, because I do not know if what I am doing is right.

Still I continue to make a flight plan.

Journal Entry: October 23, 2007

Today I actually feel the need to write to slow down my runaway emotions.

Today there is a calm about my mind, but it should frighten me.

Because I know that underneath this display of serenity lies a turbulence.

I do not want to be caught unawares when it surfaces for air or for release.

I don't even know what it is exactly.

It's deeper than a cry for help.

It's a longing of some kind.

A longing, a yearning for something old and lost.

It is succulent.

It is necessary.

I want to say it is called home, but I don't understand what that even means any more.

Is my dad's foggy world rubbing off on me?

Or am I quite simply losing my grip?

Journal Entry: December 7, 2008

I realized today as I was preparing myself to write that there was voice in my head saying,

"Today could be the day."

Today could be the day that you write something so profound, so awesome that it changes your life!

Honest to God, the voice said that to me.

And there was a time I would have listened.

But for the other voices that are louder and more obnoxious.

The *shredders* I call them.

The voices that say things like,

"Oh my God, you can't let anyone read that crap."

Shred it for God's sake.

Shred it quickly, and no one will have to know you wrote it.

Shred it, or you'll be exposed as an imposter.

Shred it blah blah blah!

Maybe I should start eating Shreddies.

To fight the shredders?

Ha ha.

I'm pretty sure the jays outside find me funny, anyway.

Journal Entry: January 16, 2009

Clearly I am not journaling as consistently as I used to.

And I can feel that this way of writing only once in a while is not particularly inspiring.

Not priming the pump of revelation at all.

But it is what it is, and if this is the only way I can write, then, so be it.

If it only helps to keep me in touch with my love of writing, that's fine, too.

Why do I feel I have to write something profound to justify writing?

Especially if my day-to-day life isn't so profound?

What is superfluous, then? My life or the attempt to write some deep meaning into it?

Honestly, I'd rather have little, useful insights once in a while than a lifestyle of constantly searching for purpose and reason.

Besides reason and purpose fly right out the window some days here.

And Dad's not even here, other than the fact

that I am so much like him, so he might as well be.

Journal entry: April 23, 2011

Long day ahead and not much time to write.

But I guard this ritual jealously and will steal a few precious moments to sit with coffee and candle-light.

Wafts of gentle cello dancing through the sleepy morning.

I hear a purr from somewhere over in the corner.

And I feel like this is my life to imagine however I choose.

For these timeless seconds, anyway.

I command this place of unimaginable imaginings, and it pleases me.

How can this not serve to uplift the day ahead?

On these self-created wings of contentment and gratitude.

Journal Questions for Part One: Identity Lost and Found

1. What are my most vivid memories of my _____, when we first met (or when I was young)?

    Don't put a time frame on this journal . . . It can be an ongoing memoir even when other questions are in process.

2. What little quirks of my _____'s do I miss most, and how do I feel when I catch a glimpse of them

again?

You may see these endearing traits surface from time to time, and it is important to acknowledge how this impacts your sense of loss over and over again. These journals are cathartic.

3. What aspects of my own nature am I glad I can bring to this situation with my _____? What aspects am I less than proud of?

Here again, remember that these journals are a conversation with yourself, and full, honest disclosure is for your eyes only.

4. How do I feel about having to give up certain activities and freedoms to care for _____?

This topic may prove difficult if shame or guilt hobbles your ability to express these feelings, but perseverance in writing about this can yield wonderful and rewarding insights.

5. What new skills do I feel I am developing through this experience with _____?

This is as empowering as a good walk or a respite break.

Journal Questions for Part Two: Dealing with Disorientation

Take at least a week to explore each question . . . even if you seem to write the same thing over and over at first. Persistent digging will eventually offer a personal insight of some kind. Journaling in this way is a type of disclosure, and as such it requires attention and sensitivity to process and accept what is coming to light.

1. What words best describe my feelings about my

   _____'s confusion?

Choose at least three feelings and write a page or two about each one.

2. As far as I can tell, what words best describe my

_____'s feelings about his/her confusion?

This is meant to bring your perception of their feelings to light.

3. What would the family think of some of these feelings?

Be specific with family members if you want, because certain individual reactions may need more attention than others—for their supportive value to you as well as critical nature.

4. What words describe my feelings about their reactions?

Remember with these journals that they are for your eyes only, so you can express whatever you need to.

Journal Questions for Part Three: Moving Past the Battle

1. What new behaviours of my _____'s make me want to scream? What nerve do they hit?

    This journaling process might need some priming and honest personal reflection, perhaps even bravery. It did for me.

2. What new behaviours or odd variations on old behaviours of my _____'s make me want to laugh, and do I allow myself to see humour in this situation? If not, why?

This may be easy for some and almost offensive for others. Alzheimer's alone is not humorous. The purpose of this journal exercise is to allow all our responses to have a voice, even if one of those voices is our own judgment.

3. When do I feel most at peace with my _____?

This may be a time of day or a particular activity, or both.

4. Can I create the circumstance for this feeling of peace to happen more?

Journal Questions for Part Four: The Ups and Downs of Finding Help

1. What feelings arise when I think about moving _____ into a home?

   Most of us know how this transition makes us feel. This journal is not so much to uncover what those feelings are, as it is to explore how we are reacting to those feelings.

2. What are other family members' feelings about this?

3. Do I feel supported by my family in the decision to move
   _____into a home?

4. What is _____ 's reaction to this move?

5. What do I like about the home that we have chosen? What
   do I not like about the home that we have chosen?

   *These are important journals, because, once we have moved our
   loved one into a home, it's easy to feel like we have lost control
   over their care. If we are going to communicate clearly with the
   caregivers there, we need to be clear within ourselves regarding
   our continuing need to protect and support this person we love.
   And it's prudent to bring praise as well as concerns to that new
   rapport.*

Journal Questions for Part Five: Finding Healing in the Journey

.

1. How has this experience changed my perspective about myself?

2. What has been the greatest insight I have had?

3. What am I most grateful for, having taken this journey with _____?

   This can be a list as long as you want. With each gratitude, we lift ourselves out of the gravity of emotions that may still be weighing on our mind.

4. What life lesson do I feel this journey has offered me?

5. If I were to write a short poem about this life lesson, what would it be called? What would it look like?

Afterword: A Silent Bugle to His Lips

In the few weeks leading up to the submission of this manuscript, I took frequent visits to a local community labyrinth. I had been enjoying this activity for some years and usually walked the path for meditation and prayer. This time though, I was seeking inspiration about the book, about my dad, about anything that could offer me strength to go the last scary lap towards the Send button on my computer.

On one particular walk, I was pondering a number of title ideas that were rolling around in my mind. One of these ideas included a turn of words that I had used to describe my dad's final moments on Christmas eve:

"A Silent bugle to his lips."

I had written it simply for its delicious sibilance, and it was one of my favourite phrases from the book itself, so I wanted to use it in a more prominent way.

The walk into the centre of the labyrinth was lovely as usual: praying, pondering, walking, listening. Then during the walk out, while still rolling this phrase around in my mind, I suddenly got stuck on the word *bugle* and couldn't stop repeating it over and over to myself. If this wasn't unusual enough I was then struck quite unexpectedly with a memory, a very vivid memory of my dad, in the last few hours of his life. I saw him lying in his bed and pawing at the air in front of him, his fingers undulating frantically up and down. I had thought at the time that he looked like he was trying to dig his way up to heaven, or out of earth, and I actually joked to him about the idea.

Now, snagged as I was on this one single word, along with the memory came a powerful insight, one that brought a flood of tears to my eyes. I saw my dad once again, lying there with this hands outstretched, fingers wiggling away in the air, and I suddenly knew with no shadow of a doubt what he had been doing.

How could I have missed it?

It was so plain to see.

Whether it was to audition his way into heaven, or summon my mom and the sweet blush on her cheeks for courage, I do not know.

But I now know this.

He was playing a bugle.

And considering how irreverently clever this wonderful man had been all his life . . . it was probably "The Last Post."

Acknowledgements:

I wish to acknowledge the tremendous support of the following women:

Susan McLean, whose initial editorial assessment of my first draft inspired me to tear it up and start again from the heart.

Mary Goy, who showed up magically when I needed magic to continue and whose experienced and generous encouragement built a bridge for me.

Sandra Owen, for her help with typing the journals in the beginning when it was too emotional for me to do so.

Dixie Peters, for her excellent work as a bereavement companion, in helping me to understand the deep mourning work I hadn't fully realized was fuelling the impulse to write this book.

And finally to my editor, Maggie Morris, who also came into my life in a most delightful and serendipitous fashion. Maggie, it seemed we were fated to work together, and I am so grateful not only for the artistic and literary skills you brought to the editing, but also for the encouraging and cheerful margin notes you offered. I truly appreciated the buoyancy they gave me.

Much thanks to all the folks at Tellwell for bringing my vision to such a professional and elegant finish. I am happy to be on board as one of your authors, and I look forward to future collaborations.

A special thanks also to my son-in-law, Matt Connell, for helping me immeasurably by creating multiple platforms of social networking for this book.

I also want to thank my many friends and family for their patience throughout the process of this writing, as well as the helpful recall many brought to some of the stories.

I especially want to thank my brother, Ronald Smith, for his constant encouragement to finish the book when it looked like I was losing steam.

A deep note of gratitude goes to the wonderful women who cared for my dad and gave me the respite I needed so badly in the last year I lived with him.

Ambre McLean, my daughter, thank you for loving and enjoying your Baba even when he was cranky. A sincere thanks for welcoming him into the circle of your celebrity nightlife. He certainly relished those moments with you.

Louise Young, my dad never hid how very fond he was of you. Thank you for the tender affection and care you so generously bestowed on him, even when he jealously insisted again and again that your lovely husband Ron was a "gink" and a "drifter" who should be disposed of.

Sare Kumagai, you are family to me. Thank you for the cheeky humour you summoned to lighten the moment every time Frankie made a pass at you!

Last, but of course not least, I want to thank my Papa, also known as my dad, also known as Frankie. It has been an honour to collect and share the many stories he told and, in so doing, to tell his story.

Notes

1. Julia Cameron, *The Artist's Way*, (New York: Jeremy P. Tarcher/Putnam, 1992), 9.

2. Inspired by the words of author, Anne Lamott: "You can either practice being right or practice being kind." "Anne Lamott>Quotes>Quotable Quotes." Goodreads.com. Copyright 2015 Goodreads Inc.

3. Online at: http://www.goodreads.com/quotes/45847-you-can-either-practice-being-right-or-practice-being-kind (accessed May 20, 2015)

4. Eudora Welty, *One Writer's Beginnings* (New York: Bookspan, 2002), 68–69.

5. Al-Anon Family Group Headquarters, Inc., preface to *Courage to Change* (New York: Al-Anon Family Group Headquarters, Inc., 1992).

6. Caring.com, "Anticipatory Grief—Coping with a Special Caregiver Stress", Copyright 2007-2015 Caring, Inc. All Rights Reserved. Excerpted with permission. Online at: https://www.caring.com/articles/anticipatory-grief-coping-with-special-caregiver-stress (accessed May 19, 2015).

Bibliography

Al-Anon Family Group Headquarters, Inc. *Courage to Change.*
New York: Al-Anon Family Group Headquarters, 1992.

Al-Anon Family Group Headquarters, Inc. *One Day at a
Time in Al-Anon.* New York: Al-Anon Family Group
Headquarters, Inc., [1968] 1990.

"Anne Lamott>Quotes>Quotable Quotes." Goodreads.com.
Copyright 2015 Goodreads Inc.

http://www.goodreads.com/quotes/45847-you-can-either-practice-being-right-or-practice-being-kind, accessed May 20, 2015.

Cameron, Julia. *The Artist's Way*. New York: Jeremy P. Tarcher/ Putnam, 1992.

Smith, Sharon Cecelia. "I Remember." *Ragged by Design*. Recorded at Kensington Studios, Toronto, 2000, Compact disc.

Spencer Scott, Paula. "Anticipatory Grief—Coping with a Special Caregiver Stress." Caring.com. Copyright 2007-2015 Caring, Inc.

https://www.caring.com/articles/anticipatory-grief-coping-with-special-caregiver-stress, accessed May 19, 2015.

Welty, Eudora. *One Writer's Beginnings*. New York: Bookspan, 2002.

Index of Images

About the Author

Sharon Cecelia Smith's long relationship with the written word has spanned a four-decade career as a singer/songwriter and performing artist.

This inaugural work marks her departure from poetic prose.

A mother of three, Sharon currently resides in Guelph, Ontario with her daughter and family.

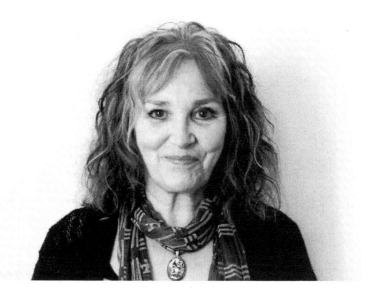

Made in the USA
Charleston, SC
23 April 2016